Fitness Doping

Jesper Andreasson · Thomas Johansson

Fitness Doping

Trajectories, Gender, Bodies and Health

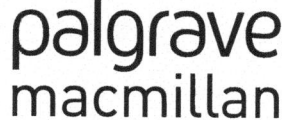

Jesper Andreasson
Department of Sport Science
Linnaeus University
Kalmar, Sweden

Thomas Johansson
Department of Education, Communication
and Learning
University of Gothenburg
Gothenburg, Sweden

ISBN 978-3-030-22104-1   ISBN 978-3-030-22105-8   (eBook)
https://doi.org/10.1007/978-3-030-22105-8

This Palgrave Macmillan imprint is published by the registered company Springer Nature Switzerland AG
The registered company address is: Gewerbestrasse 11, 6330 Cham, Switzerland

Preface

Both in research and in the public discourse, the use of illicit performance- and image-enhancing substances (PIED) has largely been connected to the context of formally governed and competitive sport. For instance, tremendous attention has been paid to cyclists, weightlifters, sprinters, and others, and scholars have discussed the different means (e.g., anabolic androgenic steroids, human growth hormones, and blood doping) elite sport athletes have used to boost their competitive edge. In the shadow of this discussion, the use of doping in the context of gym and fitness culture has largely (in comparison) proceeded unnoticed. *Fitness Doping* has been written with the intent to rectify this imbalance and take a closer look at recent developments in drug use practices in the context of gym and fitness culture.

Fitness Doping is the result of our long collaboration and our interest in the global development and growth of gym and fitness culture. We have previously published *The Global Gym. Gender, Health and Pedagogies* (2014), with Palgrave Macmillan, in which the franchising and cultural commercialization of fitness are discussed. Later, we published a second book, *Extreme Sports, Extreme Bodies. Gender, Identities and Bodies in Motion* (2019). In this second book, we took a more

carnalizing and phenomenological approach to the sports of bodybuilding, ironman triathlon, and mixed martial arts. In the volume at hand,
which is to be understood as the third and final part of the puzzle, we
have aimed to synthetize the outcomes of our previous writings and to
contribute to an ongoing debate on fitness doping, health, and gender.

In the book, we will discuss how the global development of gym and
fitness culture has impacted the general fitness doping demography in
recent decades, as well as the trajectories leading to doping and the bodily understandings/negotiations connected to the use of illicit drugs.
Clearly, it is not only bodybuilders and dedicated weightlifters who
use doping in these contexts. Initiating our work, we saw the need for
a more problematized and theoretically informed discussion on fitness
doping trajectories and the gendering of fitness doping. We are sincerely
grateful that Sharla Plant and Poppy Hull at Palgrave Macmillan, as well
as the anonymous reviewers, found our proposal interesting and relevant, making it possible for us to write and publish the book at hand.

This book builds on data that have mainly been gathered in a
Swedish context and using an ethnographic approach. In Sweden, not
only is doping prohibited in terms of trafficking, but the presence of
such substances in the body is also illegal. We have met and talked to
people operating within the context of gym and fitness culture who—in
different ways and to different extents—use doping. By generously sharing their experiences, understandings, and perspectives on things, these
people have engaged in discussions that could have legal repercussions.
We are sincerely grateful for their generosity and would like to thank all
of the women and men who took the time to talk with us and included
us in their everyday lives. We would also like to express our appreciation
to some colleagues and friends for their efforts and support. For their
role in a larger project, we would like to thank our project collabora-
tors Ellen Sverkersson, Ph.D. student at Linnaeus University, and Johan
Öhman, at the anti-doping network PRODIS (prevention of doping
in Sweden). We would also like to express our gratitude to the *Swedish
Research Council for Health, Working Life and Welfare* (FORTE) for
financial support. Thank you also to Andreas Björke and Marie Lann.

Further, we would like to thank some scholars for their input and
generous contribution in the form of reading, commenting on and

offering their insights on our work. Thank you Ask Vest Christiansen, Aarhus University, and April Henning, University of Stirling. April contributed greatly as a co-author on one of the chapters (Chapter 3). We also wish to thank Karen Williams for proof reading and editing the text. Karen, your ways with words always bring clarity to our thoughts.

Some chapters in the book build on articles previously published by the authors in academic journals, including *Sport in Society*, *Performance Enhancement and Health*, *Journal of Sport and Social Issues* and *Social Sciences*.

Kalmar, Sweden   Jesper Andreasson
Gothenburg, Sweden   Thomas Johansson
May 2019

Contents

Part I

Contextualizing Fitness Doping

1

Introduction

Introduction

In the research, and as a phenomenon, the use of illicit performance- and image-enhancing drugs (PIED), such as anabolic androgenic steroids (henceforth steroids) and human growth hormones, has commonly been understood as either a concern for formally governed competitions in (elite) sports (i.e., 'sport doping') or a public health issue—thus, as a social/societal problem (Dimeo, 2007; Waddington, 2000). Tremendous investments have been made in researching drug use practices in relation to organized elite sports and how doping can be prevented to ensure the maintenance of highly held ideals concerning fair play (Waddington & Smith, 2009). In recent decades, however, scholars have increasingly recognized doping as both a societal problem and a public health issue (Brennan, Wells & van Hout, 2017; Christiansen, 2018; Van Hout & Hearne, 2016), and it has primarily been associated with strength training at various gyms, and within gym, and fitness culture per se.

It has often been suggested that the social impact of the gym and fitness environment, that is, the kind of mentality nourished and the socialization process occurring there, is key to understanding drug use outside the

© The Author(s) 2020
J. Andreasson and T. Johansson, *Fitness Doping*,
https://doi.org/10.1007/978-3-030-22105-8_1

sphere of formally governed sports. In the late 1970s and early 1980s when gym and fitness culture expanded significantly (Andreasson & Johansson, 2014), reports also began to surface that recreational fitness doping had gained popularity among young people, as a means of increasing muscle size and improving physical appearance, among other things (Parkinson & Evans, 2006; Sas-Nowosielski, 2006). Initial discussions in the research and in the public discourse came to focus on male bodybuilders, their risk behavior, and their willingness to experiment with all sorts of substances in their pursuit of muscles and masculinity (Gaines & Butler, 1974; Klein, 1993; Monaghan, 2001). The cultural studies literature largely described the development of an underground phenomenon and culture, in which bodybuilding men (and some women) used doping to create extraordinary bodies, which were displayed in front of cheering audiences at bodybuilding competitions, or for that matter in front of mirrors at the gym.

Gradually acquiring the status of a mass leisure activity, however, gym and fitness culture has changed, as has the image of the gym since the 1970s (Smith Maguire, 2008). Today, all around the world, people are using these facilities to exercise their bodies and achieve success and health in everyday life (Andreasson & Johansson, 2014). In this 'new' culture, the highest goals and aspirations are commercialized and framed in terms of youth and health, and the modern fitness center is seen or displayed as a health clinic for 'the masses' (Sassatelli, 2010). Paradoxically, concurrently with cultural fitness trends and the idealization of an active and healthy life, the emphasis placed on the body and its appearance has contributed to persistent doping problems.

Although it is still the case that doping practices in this context are mainly connected to the art and sport of bodybuilding, the fitness geography is changing, and so is the doping demography. With little hope of fame or financial gain, non-competitive bodybuilders as well as 'regular' gymgoers are increasingly engaging in drug use practices (Locks & Richardson, 2012). Little by little, women have also entered the realm of fitness doping (Jespersen, 2012; McGrath & Chananie-Hill, 2009; Van Hout & Hearne, 2016). Thus, boosted by an increasing focus on and preoccupation with body image issues among both men and women (Andreasson & Johansson, 2014; Cash & Pruzinsky, 2002), the widespread availability of doping, and the growing prevalence among mainstream fitness groups internationally, the use of doping is still considered a growing public health issue in many Western societies (Christiansen, 2018; Van Hout & Hearne, 2016).

The global development of gym and fitness culture (which we will return to in Chapter 2) has been remarkable and parallels even more widespread processes of medialization and medicalization in Western societies. Extreme and muscular bodies are visualized in popular media, and bodies are trained and molded with the help of high-tech machines, or through franchised and commercially driven training programs. Different products (licit and illicit) have been developed to further boost performance and efforts to achieve fame. Largely, but not exclusively, all these processes boil down to one thing, the body, and how it is to be understood as a contemporary modern phenomenon. Thus, we live in an era of bodies in motion, of performance, muscles, swelling veins, and dreams of the right bodily proportions. Within gym and fitness culture, there has been a revolution of technologies of the self, and extending beyond this cultural context, people's ways of relating to and understanding the body in contemporary society have changed noticeably during a relatively short period of time. This is not only a story about the development of tools and techniques to shape and show human flesh through exercise. Rather, it is about bodies that are in constant transformation through training, diets, plastic surgery, and the use of licit and sometimes illicit drugs. It is a story about the gradual emergence of a new gaze and way to relate to the human body. Fueled by the development of gym and fitness culture, among other things, the body has come to be perceived as plastic and ever transgressive. Largely, at the core of gym and fitness culture, we thus find a story about a body in becoming.

The development within gym and fitness culture originated from a subcultural and masculine phenomenon. Icons such as Arnold Schwarzenegger, and earlier Eugen Sandow, exemplified how muscles, masculinity, and extreme bodies were made. Today, however, gym and fitness culture have transformed and become an arena for transforming bodies and gender transgressions. The 1990s is something of a dividing line, when female bodybuilders started to challenge public conceptions of binary gender configurations. Bodies are made at the gym, but so is gender. Consequently, women's gradual integration has helped rewrite the gender of fitness culture, and from being an almost exclusively masculine culture, this arena for working out has diversified in relation to gender, age, and ethnicity. Like a hub in this development of a particular body culture, *the fitness revolution* (Andreasson & Johansson, 2014), we find the promotion of an interest in developing the body, cherishing its abilities and performance, and its beauty. The question of health and balance is clearly present, but so is the negotiable line that is sometimes drawn between health, on the one hand, and excessive training, bodily disorders, and unhealthy lifestyles, including the use of doping, on the other.

Aims and Methodological Point of Departure

Within the context of recent developments in gym and fitness culture, the aim of this book is twofold. *First*, we aim to investigate and identify different processes through which a person becomes a 'fitness doper,' that is, the trajectories leading to doping. There is currently surprisingly little scholarship available that involves qualitative research on young people's doping trajectories in this cultural context. To prevent doping, we need to understand the norms, ideas, and networks of people who engage in it, even though they (at least to some extent) are aware that there are risks and potential health costs associated with the practice. To develop effective prevention methods, we also need to understand the longitudinal processes through which the practice gradually becomes an option for the individual.

In the book, we will address these issues and try to move forward our understanding of and the debate on fitness doping trajectories. We will not only focus on doping use in relation to strength-training activities, traditionally dominated by young men, but also analyze how it is understood by people who belong to other demographic fitness groups or who specialize in other kinds of exercise within this culture, such as group training activities. Therefore, and *second*, we also aim to problematize and possibly challenge the gender politics that have traditionally been attached to fitness doping. Analytically, we will pay attention to processes through which distinctions between masculinity/femininity, criminal/legal, and healthy/unhealthy bodies are negotiated and destabilized by users, both online and away from the keyboard. The overall aims will be addressed by posing the following research questions:

- In what ways can different fitness doping trajectories and the processes of becoming and unbecoming a fitness doper be understood?
- In what ways are the processes and cultural patterns of socialization and learning regarding fitness doping affected by demographic variables, such as gender, lifestyle, and age?
- In what ways is fitness doping discussed, negotiated, and legitimized/normalized in the context of online communication and communities?
- What kinds of perspectives on health, physical training, the body, and lifestyles do fitness dopers adopt, and how are drug use practices related to these perspectives?
- What does a changing fitness doping demography entail as regards future challenges and implications in the research and in relation to existing anti-doping work and prevention strategies?

To address the above questions and aims, we have utilized a qualitative mixed methods approach, consisting of qualitative biographical interviews, observations, Internet material from online communications, and an overall ethnographic approach to the research (Fangen, 2005; Hammersley & Atkinson, 1995). As part of a larger project, the empirical material used can be said to derive from two datasets. *First*, we have conducted a longitudinal ethnographic study in which more than 30 fitness dopers have been repeatedly interviewed and followed over time, in training and everyday life. *Second*, we have looked into the ways in which doping is perceived and negotiated socially in the specific sociocultural context of an Internet-mediated, open online community called Flashback. In this community, anyone with an Internet connection can learn about doping and comment on their experience and knowledge of it. In our sampling of postings, we have primarily focused on themes connected to doping, in general, and fitness doping trajectories, gender, and health, in particular. In our analysis, these two datasets have been treated and understood as tightly interwoven and guided by the shared, overall aims, as outlined above (see Chapter 10 for further information on methodology and method).

Although the book takes an international approach to fitness doping, our data have mainly been gathered in a Swedish context, which calls for some initial comments. For example, the Swedish Doping Act (1991:1969), adopted in 1991, prohibits not only the possession and trafficking of doping, but also the presence of doping substances in the body. Since the 1990s, fitness doping has been associated with increasingly strict penalties and comprehensive anti-doping campaigns. To this end, and in an international comparison, fitness doping in Sweden can reasonably be understood as a marginalized cultural practice. We will return to this discussion on national variations in fitness doping policy and practice in Chapter 3.

Concepts and Terminology

Engaging in research on doping inevitably means becoming involved in morally loaded discourses (Christiansen, 2018). Within the formally governed sport context, for example, the ban on doping has been constructed in line with strong desires to ensure the value, spirit, and integrity of modern sport, building on the ideal that winning should be the result of honest excellence in performance, and nothing else (Beamish & Ritchie 2007, p. 105). Thus, cheaters in sport have been harshly condemned in the public discourse. In addition, in the gym and fitness context, doping has been described/analyzed in terms of deviance, marginalization, and destructive masculinities (Klein, 1993; Monaghan, 2001). Put differently, when discussing and researching doping, we are entering a specific social and cultural landscape in which our use of concepts and terminology is of great importance.

When talking about *doping* broadly in this book, we are primarily referring to activities banned by national legislation, including the use, possession, and/or selling of prohibited substances, such as steroids and human growth hormones (Lindholm, 2013). Discussing the use of doping may also be connected to the World Anti-Doping Agency (WADA), whose goal is to protect athletes' health and safeguard the notion of fair play. Because it operates outside the sport context, however, this organization has a limited impact on doping use in the gym and fitness context.

As a means of stressing the contextual differences between doping in sport and doping in gym and fitness culture, terms such as 'vanity doping,' 'fitness doping,' 'recreational doping,' and the use of 'performance- and image-enhancing drugs' (PIED) have sometimes been employed in the gym and fitness context (see, e.g., Christiansen, 2009; Thualagant, 2012). So as not to predetermine the motives underlying different pathways to and from doping, we have chosen to employ the term *fitness doping*. We also talk about doping using the terms PIEDs. We have made these choices with the intent to explicitly emphasize the cultural context (fitness culture) of the form of doping in question and to, at the same time, not try to pinpoint the reasons for doping (see also, Andreasson, 2015).

Regarding terminology, we prefer the term 'use' for describing our participants' practices, as opposed to the concepts of 'misuse' and 'abuse,' both of which are contested by scholars and morally loaded (Christiansen, Schmidt Vinther & Liokaftos, 2016, p. 2). Our goal here is to maintain an ethnographic approach to the research presentation, as we consider 'use' to be more reflective of the data gathered (cf. WHO, 2015). This does not mean, however, that we are denying that fitness doping may lead to or cause severe side effects in the form of physical and mental health problems. Although not the focus of this book, we are fully aware of the diverse documented side effects connected to the use of PIEDs, including increases in aggressive behavior and depression, acne, hair loss, disruption of growth, and damage to tendons, ligaments as well as the liver (ACMD, 2010; Kimegård, 2015). Furthermore, for women there is a risk of deepening of the voice, clitoris enlargement, menstruation irregularities, and reduced fertility, and for men, we also see gynecomastia, testicular atrophy, and erectile dysfunction (Evans-Brown, McVeigh, Perkins & Bellis, 2012). We are also aware that these side effects should be understood as dose related and to some extent dependent on how knowledgeable and familiar a user may be with different kinds of substances, and whether or not he/she seeks medical advice if needed.

Fitness Doping Prevalence

Although scholars have mainly focused on doping in sport (Dimeo & Møller, 2018; Mottram, 2006; Waddington & Smith 2009), there are also numerous studies of doping and drug use in the gym and fitness context (Christiansen, 2018; Kimegård, 2015; Monaghan, 2012). The results from these studies, however, present a somewhat scattered picture, and the extent of use is thought to vary greatly (Bergsgard, Tangen, Barland & Breivik, 1996; Brennan, Wells & van Hout, 2017; Pedersen, 2010). For example, a study on steroid use conducted in Cyprus showed that 11.6% of the young people at 22 gyms reported using prohibited substances for performance- and image-enhancing purposes (Kartakoullis, Phellas, Pouloukas, Petrou & Loizou, 2008), whereas in Sweden these figures seem to be lower, with 4% of women and 5% of men at fitness centers reporting personal experiences of fitness doping use (Hoff, 2013; Swedish National Institute of Public Health, 2011). The cultural context of gym and fitness has also been emphasized in the research, and in a survey conducted among gym members at 18 gyms in the United Arab Emirates, Al-Falasi, Al-Dahmani, and Al-Eisaei (2008) concluded that as many as 59% of participants believed that the risks of using steroids were outweighed by the possible benefits of the drugs. There are also studies indicating that fitness doping is decreasing. A US-based annual youth survey, for example, suggests that lifetime steroid use dropped to 1.2% in 2017, from being nearly three times as high at the beginning of the millennium (Johnston et al., 2018; Pope et al., 2014). In conclusion, our understanding of and research on the historical development of PIED use in the fitness context is not conclusive and to some extent still fairly rudimentary.

There are of course manifold explanations for why existing knowledge is limited regarding fitness doping prevalence and practices. *First*, standardized indicators have not proven to be fully reliable in measuring the percentage of doping users in a given population, whether it concerns sport doping or fitness doping, or any other forms of doping use for that matter (Christiansen, 2018). *Second*, traditional surveys have often been used to gather information on the extent of use in different countries, but just as in other research on sensitive and potentially stigmatizing topics, there are typically low response rates and underreporting, which may make it difficult to draw conclusions regarding, in this case, use of doping in the general population in a given country. *Thirdly*, we are dealing with a growing arena of online communication in which the handling and trafficking of drugs operate on a supranational rather than national level. In relation to this, researchers, as well as authorities, have found it challenging to grasp and once and for all define a clear sampling pool. This also relates to the fact that doping can be viewed as an umbrella term for a wide range of substances, some of which may be licit in certain countries but illicit in others. Therefore, it is not obvious that researchers and respondents understand the terminology used in the same way (see European Commission, 2014), although they may well understand whether the practice is accepted or viewed as a criminal or marginalized practice in a given society or context.

Analytical Framework

One important theme and focus of this book is the relation between the more subcultural phenomenon of bodybuilding, fitness doping and extreme bodies, and the more general approach to the body found in gym and fitness culture. What we are trying to elaborate on is the relation between a more 'deviant' and criminal activity and lifestyle, and the more common and normalized practice of using different means to promote a specific body ideal. This theme will be present throughout the book, and we will pay extra attention to how fitness dopers talk about, understand, and negotiate this relation. We have chosen to elaborate on this using the concept of subculture, and its relation to what can be considered hegemonic culture, that is, the sociocultural context and understanding of everyday life that is embraced by most people in society. We are, of course, aware that this distinction is difficult to make, and our intention is not to define once and for all where the line between the particular and the general should be drawn, but rather to use this gestalt as an intriguing and exciting point of departure.

In theories of subcultures, we often find a more or less clear distinction between subculture and *mainstream* or *common culture*. There is, of course, a varyingly complex relationship between what is 'sub-' and what is dominant or hegemonic (Johansson & Herz, 2019). Subcultures are frequently spectacular, but there is also a strong affinity between everyday culture and different subcultures (Baker, Robards & Buttigieg, 2015). The visibility, distinctness, and desire expressed in subcultural communities serve to recruit people to these kinds of subgroups. The perspectives on subcultures have also varied over time. According to Hebdige (1979), for example, subcultures are implacably incorporated into and consumed by mainstream culture. At the same time, and in contrast, Hodkinson (2002) argued that there is often a high level of distinctiveness, stability, and durability—in the sense of collective identity—fostered within subcultures. Thus, what we are studying here is the relationship between common and general sociocultural patterns in society and the more specific and distinct sociocultural patterns, communities, and lifestyles in which fitness doping is included. Naturally, defining mainstream or common culture is almost impossible. In a similar vein, what is regarded as subcultural varies greatly. Given this, we must be satisfied with trying to grapple with and understand the ongoing and changing relationship between more general and more specific sociocultural patterns in society.

A closer look at specific subcultures provides a clearer picture of their importance in relation to changing subjectivities (Johansson, Andreasson & Mattsson, 2017). In particular, we can see how subcultures are intimately interwoven with and tied into societal and cultural transformations. For example, ever since the 1970s, bodybuilding has been successively transforming into fitness. In this respect, it has gradually moved in the direction of becoming mainstream. The core values of the hard—bodybuilding—body, focused on muscle training, health, and asceticism, are, for example, very prominent in the contemporary fitness culture, as well as in the more common, dominant sociocultural patterns observed in many Western countries. What is interesting here is the process through which common culture gradually incorporates certain lifestyle attributes and values of the subculture of bodybuilding. Body techniques, discipline, and knowledge about how to transform the body are being transformed, marketed, and commercialized. Yet certain bodies are still labeled as 'too' extreme—that is, connected to unhealthy lifestyles, drugs, and narcissism—and are thus being marginalized from the more public domains of gym and fitness culture. The intricate interplay between the subculture and the processes of mainstreaming is a central mechanism in contemporary fitness culture. Some aspects of body ideals and lifestyles are incorporated into more general cultural trends, while other aspects are not.

If we explore the relationship between subcultures and the mainstreaming of certain values, opinions, and practices, it becomes apparent that certain subcultural values and sentiments gradually, and over time, tend to become normalized, accepted, and routinized ways of relating to, for example, the body, health, politics, and societal values. Subcultural expressions and styles become significant and worth studying when they affect the balance between what is subcultural and what is 'common.' Listening to people's voices, narratives, and expressions also reveals micro-transformations of the subjective content found in subcultures and society. Looking more closely at the social-psychological and cultural level in relation to these fundamental societal changes also leads us to interesting analyses of how the more ephemeral aspects of subcultures—such as styles, clothes, values, and artifacts—can be understood as parts of more general transformations in society. At the same time, subcultures seem to—on a regular basis—recreate and reinvent themselves. This is also part of the fascination and desire involved in the constant interplay between subcultures and society, between 'the extreme' and 'the normal,' health and unhealth, as well as the criminal and legal.

This discussion of subcultures will be used as a way into the book. Adding to this, we will use other conceptual tools in the chapters—for example, *gender* and the concept of *role exit*. We prefer to introduce and explain these in the chapters where they are set in motion. Further, we will also develop our own theoretical lens and toolbox throughout the book, allowing us to suggest new conceptual approaches to addressing the relationship between subculture and common culture, which has been prominent in doping studies. Having said this, we will now turn to the structure and content of the book.

Readers' Guidelines

In its presentation, the book has been divided into four parts. The first part consists of three chapters (1–3) and is intended to introduce and contextualize the subject matter broadly. In this introductory chapter, we have explained the general context and aims of the book, as well as the data underlying the results. We have also addressed some conceptual choices made and the theoretical and analytical framework from which the book starts out. In Chapter 2, we present an extended discussion of the historical development of gym and fitness culture, in general, and contemporary perspectives on fitness doping, in particular. This first substantial chapter is intended to frame the purposes of the book historically and culturally. In Chapter 3, we address fitness doping in a comparative manner, investigating how fitness doping can be understood in relation to, and how it is affected by, different national contexts and welfare state regimes. Situated within the context of a globalized and glocalized gym and fitness culture, we conduct a comparative analysis, focusing on fitness doping in relation to policy, practice, and prevention in the USA and Sweden. Here, we also address the complex interplay between various supranational structures and global systems of anti-doping work and campaigns, on the one hand, and diverse local implementations of prevention policies and the development of national fitness doping cultures, communities, and practices, on the other.

The second and third part of the book constitutes the main empirical contribution, and it is here we explicitly address our twofold aim. The second part, *Doping Trajectories*, consists of Chapters 4–6. In Chapter 4, we let the reader become acquainted with some of the men and women who have generously shared their experiences and views. Through personal portraits in the form of case studies, we describe a number of fitness dopers and their trajectories to fitness doping, as well as their perspectives on training, muscles, gender, and more. In Chapter 5, we develop the discussion initiated in previous chapters on doping trajectories and employ a cultural and sociological perspective, focusing on the processes of becoming and unbecoming a fitness doping user, and how doping is negotiated in relation to ideas and ideals concerning health, gender, Swedish law, and thoughts about individual freedom, among other things. Here, we also consider the question of sporting background and fitness dopers' initiation into gym and fitness training. In Chapter 6, we focus on how fitness doping is perceived and negotiated socially in the context of an Internet-mediated, online community. Here, we are interested in the ways in which the risks and health costs associated with drug use practices are negotiated, and in how ideas about the 'genetic max,' as well as the ultimate possibility of exceeding one's limits and creating something special and extraordinary, circulate in the imaginary world of online muscle-building and drug use practices.

The third part of the book, *Doped Bodies and Gender*, consists of Chapters 7 and 8. In Chapter 7, we describe the gendering of doped bodies in the fitness doping research. Specifically, we focus on the kind of masculinity that historically has been attached to our understanding of the reasons for fitness doping. Here, we dissect and analyze the construction of masculinity and drug use practices in gym and fitness culture. We discuss how our participants in some ways conform to gender fantasies that rest on binary understandings of gendered, doped bodies, but also how different negotiations and inclusive subversions of traditional gender norms are manifested in male users' narratives and in online communication. In Chapter 8, we also use both interview material and data from various postings on a pro-doping online community, but here, the focus is on female fitness dopers and how they understand and negotiate their use in relation to gender and the body. In the chapter, we discuss to what extent women are increasingly invited to and have become more integrated into a fitness (doping) community and subculture, and the consequences this inclusion may have.

Finally, in the fourth part of the book, *Conclusions*, we bring the threads together in a concise manner. In Chapter 9, we explicitly address the aims of the book and present some concluding thoughts on fitness doping trajectories and the gendering of fitness doping. Here, we also, in a more speculative vein, approach the question of how a changing fitness culture and doping demography are related to current and future developments in fitness doping and doping prevention. This part also contains Chapter 10, in which we explain the research design and methodology of the project(s) on which the book is based.

References

ACMD. (2010). *Consideration of the anabolic steroids.* London: Home Office.

Al-Falasi, O., Al-Dahmani, K., & Al-Eisaei, K. (2008). Knowledge, attitude and practice of anabolic steroids use among gym users in Al-Ain District, United Arab Emirates. *The Open Sports Medicine Journal, 9*(2), 75–81.

Andreasson, J. (2015). Reconceptualising the gender of fitness doping: Performing and negotiating masculinity through drug-use practices. *Social Sciences, 4,* 546–562.

Andreasson, J., & Johansson, T. (2014). *The global gym: Gender, health and pedagogies.* Basingstoke, UK: Palgrave Macmillan.

Baker, S., Robards, B., & Buttigieg, B. (2015). *Youth cultures and subcultures: Australian perspectives.* Farnham, UK: Ashgate.

Beamish, R., & Ritchie, I. (2007). *Fastest, highest, strongest: A critique of high-performance sport.* London and New York: Routledge.

Bergsgard, N.-A., Tangen, J.-O., Barland, B., & Breivik, G. (1996). Doping in norwegian gyms—A big problem? *International Review for Sociology of Sport, 34*(4), 351–364.

Brennan, R., Wells, J., & van Hout, M. C. (2017). The injecting use of image and performance-enhancing drugs (IPED) in the general population: A systematic review. *Health and Social Care in the Community, 25*(5), 1459–1531.

Cash, T., & Pruzinsky, T. (2002). *Body image: A handbook of theory, research, and clinical practice.* New York, NY: Guildford Press.

Christiansen, A. V. (2009). Doping in fitness and strength training environments: Politics, motives and masculinity. In V. Møller, M. McNamme, & P. Dimeo (Eds.), *Elite sport, doping and public health.* Odense: University Press of Southern Denmark.

Christiansen, A. V. (2018). *Motionsdoping. Styrketræning, identitet og kultur* [Recreational doping: Strength training, identity and culture]. Aarhus, Denmark: Aarhus Universitetsforlag.

Christiansen, A. V., Schmidt Vinther, A., & Liokaftos, D. (2016). Outline of a typology of men's use of anabolic androgenic steroids in fitness and strength training environments. *Drugs: Education, Prevention and Policy.* https://doi.org/10.1080/09687637.2016.1231173.

Dimeo, P. (2007). *A history of drug use in sport 1876–1976: Beyond good and evil.* London and New York: Routledge.

Dimeo, P., & Møller, V. (2018). *The anti-doping crisis in sport: Causes, consequences, solutions.* London: Routledge.

European Commission. (2014). *Study on doping prevention: A map of legal, regulatory and prevention practice provisions in EU 28.* Luxembourg: Publications Office of the European Union.

Evans-Brown, M., McVeigh, J., Perkins, C., & Bellis, M. A. (2012). *Human enhancement drugs: The emerging challenges to public health.* Liverpool: North West Public Health Observatory.

Fangen, K. (2005). *Deltagande observation* [Participant observation]. Malmö: Liber.

Gaines, C., & Butler, G. (1974). *Pumping iron: The art and sport of bodybuilding.* London: Sphere Books Ltd.

Hammersley, M., & Atkinson, P. (1995). *Ethnography: Principles in practice.* London: Routledge.

Hebdige, D. (1979). *Subculture: The meaning of style.* London: Routledge.

Hodkinson, P. (2002). *Goth: Identity, style and subculture.* Oxford: Berg.

Hoff, D. (2013). Dopning utanför idrotten – individualisering och muskulösa skönhetsideal. En studie av dopning i grundskola, gymnasium och på gym i Kalmar kommun. *Scandinavian Sport Studies Forum, 4,* 1–24.

Jespersen, M. R. (2012). "Definitely not for women": An online community's reflections on women's use of performance enhancing drugs. In J. Tolleneer, S. Sterckz, & P. Bonte (Eds.), *Athletic enhancement, human nature and ethics: Threats and opportunities of doping technologies* (pp. 201–218). Dordrecht, The Netherlands: Springer.

Johansson, T., Andreasson, J., & Mattsson, C. (2017). From subcultures to common culture: Bodybuilders, skinheads, and the normalization of the marginal. *Sage Open, 7*(2), 1–9.

Johansson, T., & Herz, M. (2019). *Youth studies in transition: Culture, generation and new learning processes.* Springer. Forthcoming.

Johnston, L. D., Miech, R. A., O'Malley, P. M., Bachman, J. G., Schulenberg, J. E., & Patrick, M. E. (2018). *Monitoring the future national survey results on drug use: 1975–2017—Overview, key findings on adolescent drug use.* Ann Arbor: Institute for Social Research, The University of Michigan.

Kartakoullis, N. L., Phellas, C., Pouloukas, S., Petrou, M., & Loizou, C. (2008). The use of anabolic steroids and other prohibited substances by gym enthusiasts in Cyprus. *International Review for the Sociology of Sport, 43*(3), 271–287.

Kimegård, A. (2015). A qualitative study of anabolic steroid use amongst gym users in the United Kingdom: Motives, beliefs and experiences. *Journal of Substance Use, 20*(4), 288–294.

Klein, A. (1993). *Little big men: Bodybuilding, subculture and gender construction.* New York: State University of New York Press.

Lindholm, J. (2013). Does legislating against doping in sports make sense? Comparing Sweden and the United States suggest not. *Virginia Sports & Entertainment Law Journal, 13*(1), 21–34.

Locks, A., & Richardson, N. (2012). *Critical readings in bodybuilding.* London: Routledge.

McGrath, S., & Chananie-Hill, R. (2009). 'Big Freaky-Looking Women': Normalizing gender transgression through bodybuilding. *Sociology of Sport Journal, 26,* 235–254.

Monaghan, L. F. (2001). *Bodybuilding, drugs and risk: Health, risk and society.* New York: Routledge.

Monaghan, L. F. (2012). Accounting for illicit steroid use: Bodybuilders' justifications. In A. Locks & N. Richardson (Eds.), *Critical readings in bodybuilding.* New York: Routledge.

Mottram, D. R. (Ed.). (2006). *Drugs in sport* (4th ed.). London and New York: Routledge.

Parkinson, A. B., & Evans, N. A. (2006). Anabolic androgenic steroids: A survey of 500 users. *Medicine and Science in Sport and Exercise, 38*(4), 644–651.

Pedersen, I. K. (2010). Doping and the perfect body expert: Social and cultural indicators of performance-enhancing drug use in Danish gyms. *Sport in Society: Cultures, Commerce, Media, Politics, 13*(3), 503–516.

Pope, H. G., Kanayama, G., Athey, A., Ryan, E., Hudson, J. I., & Baggish, A. (2014). The lifetime prevalence of anabolic-androgenic steroid use and dependence in Americans: Current best estimates. *The American Journal on Addictions, 23*(4), 371–377.

Sas-Nowosielski, K. (2006). The abuse of anabolic-androgenic steroids by Polish school-aged adolescents. *Biology of Sport, 23*(3), 225–235.

Sassatelli, R. (2010). *Fitness culture: Gyms and the commercialisation of discipline and fun.* Hampshire: Palgrave Macmillan.

Smith Maguire, J. (2008). *Fit for consumption. Sociology and the business of fitness.* London and New York: Routledge.

Swedish National Institute of Public Health. (2011). *Dopning i Samhället* [Doping in society]. Östersund, Sweden: Statens Folkhälsoinstitut.

The Swedish Doping Act. (1991:1969). *Dopningslagen.* Stockholm, Sweden: Svensk författningssamling SFS.

Thualagant, N. (2012). The conceptualization of fitness doping and its limitations. *Sport in Society: Cultures, Commerce, Media, Politics, 15*(3), 409–419.

Van Hout, M. C., & Hearne, E. (2016). Netnography of female use of the synthetic growth hormone CJC-1295: Pulses and potions. *Substance Use & Misuse.* https://doi.org/10.3109/10826084.2015.1082595.

Waddington, I. (2000). *Sport, health and drugs: A critical sociological perspective.* London and New York: Routledge.

Waddington, I., & Smith, A. (2009). *An introduction to drugs in sport: Addicted to winning?.* London and New York: Routledge.

WHO. (2015). Lexicon of alcohol and drug terms published by the World Health Organization. WHO. Retrieved from http://www.who.int/substance_abuse/terminology/who_lexicon/en/.

2

Doping—Historical and Contemporary Perspectives

Introduction

With promises of new technologies, and the use of biochemical resources to boost performance and muscle mass, doping has been historically, and still is, intertwined with the development of modern organized sport. The history of doping is thus also one of sport, modernity and the plastic and changeable body. Through hegemonic ideas/ideals about performing bodies, different sports have successively been modernized since the mid-1800s (Dimeo, 2007), and within this modernization process, we also find the use of performance- and image-enhancing drugs (PIEDs). In the 1930s, for example, different kinds of drugs were used to combat fatigue and increase performance. This was largely done in a more or less discredited manner, especially in comparison with contemporary perspectives on doping in the public discourse. Monkey gland extracts, sodium phosphates, amphetamine, and sugary sweets were used frequently at this time. Steroids were also widely used by Soviet weightlifters and American bodybuilders (among others) in the 1950s (Dimeo, 2007; see also Connolly, 2015). Consequently, PIED use was to some extent understood as part of a medical and scientific approach to the performing, muscular,

© The Author(s) 2020
J. Andreasson and T. Johansson, *Fitness Doping*,
https://doi.org/10.1007/978-3-030-22105-8_2

and competent body (Holt, Iouletta, & Sönksen, 2009). It is unclear whether the doctors and policymakers in, for example, East Germany and other countries had knowledge about the potential side effects and health risks associated with the use of different drugs (Dimeo & Hunt, 2011). Gradually, however, reports on health problems became more frequent.

The use of steroids and, more broadly, prohibited doping substances in a sport context has been a subject of debate for decades. Still, and as touched on in the previous chapter, many studies have indicated that one main reason for people commencing with these drugs is muscle-building and image-enhancing, and as such, it is closely related to the development of gym and fitness culture (Petrocelli, Oberweis, & Petrocelli, 2008; Evans-Brown, McVeigh, Perkins, & Belli, 2012). In relation to the global development and expansion of gym and fitness culture, for example, the use of PIEDs among gym members has been reported in a number of countries in Europe (Hoff, 2013; Kimegård, 2015; Christiansen, 2018), North America (Pope et al., 2014), Brazil (Santos, Da Rocha, & Da Silva, 2011), the United Arab Emirates (Al-Falasi, Al-Dahmani, & Al-Eisaei, 2008), and Iran (Allahverdipour, Jalilian, & Shaghaghi, 2012), to name a few. Thus, PIED use in the gym population would seem to present a challenge to public health on a global scale. Although recognized in research as well as by central stakeholders, nationally as well as internationally, the worldwide trade in and use of doping substances, in general and in contrast to the continuous refinement of anti-doping organizations and work, have continued to increase over time (Antonopoulos & Hall, 2016). Furthermore, despite the predominant role played by the Internet in the distribution of PIEDs, little is known about the online supply and global distribution of doping products in contemporary societies (Pineau et al., 2016).

In this chapter, we will take a closer look at the historical development of gym and fitness culture, in general, and the use of PIEDs (fitness doping) in this context, in particular. We will present a framework that can be used to analyze changing attitudes, views, and practices related to PIED use. We will distinguish between four historical phases. In the *first phase*, we find optimism and increasing levels of PIED use, culminating in the creation of a bodybuilding subculture in the *second phase*. Thereafter follows a critical *third phase*, where steroids are gradually seen as morally objectionable.

In the late 1980s and early 1990s, we see an increasing moral judgment of bodybuilders and the widespread use of doping as a means to achieve the genetic max. The *fourth phase*, The Fitness Revolution, can be seen as a transformational phase in the entire gym culture, characterized by great changes in body and coaching ideals. In this phase, the huge bodybuilding body is replaced with the well-defined and moderately muscular fitness body. But what impact have these changes (had) on fitness doping practices during the twenty-first century? At the end of the chapter, we will speculate about the possible development of a *fifth phase*, and what that could bring.

The Pre-history of Gym Culture and Doping

> The extensive use of medicinal products for the alleviation of the symptoms of disease can be traced back to the Greek physician, Galen, in the third century BC. Interestingly, it was Galen who reported that ancient Greek athletes used stimulants to enhance their physical performance. [...] In Roman times, gladiators used stimulants to maintain energy levels after injury. Similar behaviour by medieval knights has also been noted. (Verroken, 2006, p. 29)

Like the alchemists' quest for the magic formula to make gold, there are examples of people throughout history searching for a 'magic' potion that will give them a competitive edge and a shortcut to their goals. As suggested above, the use of PIEDs can be traced all the way back to the values regarding and approaches to the physically competent body and the hegemonic body ideals found in ancient Greece and Rome. A more contemporary period in the history of fitness doping, however, is the early 1900s and what has been called the development of *physical culture*.

Located mainly in the USA, the growth of physical culture brought with it new techniques for forming and developing a strong, muscular, and masculine body (Budd, 1997). Influenced by the Swedish, Danish, and German gymnastic movements, scientists in the USA, and internationally, gradually turned their focus and interest to physical education and methods of improving human health and strength (Andreasson & Johansson, 2014a). The physical culture movement was strongly supported by physicians, who regarded physical culture, especially among men, as a way to combat degeneration and the weakening of public health and the nation. At this time, physical culture enthusiasts and the medical establishment did not encourage excessive muscular development. The ordination was for gymnastics and hygienic moderation, rather than for building muscles (Vertinsky, 1999).

When strong man Eugen Sandow, usually referred to as one of the founding fathers of bodybuilding, arrived in America in 1893, he was immediately criticized and laughed at. Sensing the attitudes and fashion of the time, Sandow did not market himself as the world's strongest man, but as the world's most developed and/or perfect man. Thus, the attention was shifted partly from strength and muscles to the look of the male physique, which increasingly made the practice of physical culture, the body and the image of the body into a marketable commodity (Budd, 1997). The medical profession was even more critical of Bernarr Mac-Fadden, the father of physical culture, calling him a narcissist. Members of the respectable medical profession saw MacFadden as an expression of the subversion of respectability, and as a threat to the 'natural' boundaries between masculinity and femininity.

The status of muscular bodies gradually changed, however. Early bodybuilding competitions in the 1930s and 1940s were meant as public demonstrations of what bodybuilding could do to reverse the corrosive effects of modern civilization (Liokaftos, 2018). Emphasis was initially put on displaying the 'natural body.' Notions such as ease, grace, and naturalness were central to the participants' success as models. Gradually, however, classical ideals of Apollonian perfection in accord with ideals from ancient Greece were eroded and replaced with mahogany tanned bodies formed on California beaches. In the late 1950s and 1960s, PIEDs were also introduced in bodybuilding. At this time, doctors and the medical profession were not critical of muscular bodies. On the contrary, there was a growing fascination with the technological advances. In contrast to the medical profession's skepticism about muscular male bodies at the end of the nineteenth century, muscular male bodies were now regarded as a sign of progress and of successful scientific control of the body and its growth.

At the 1954 World Weightlifting Championships in Vienna, Austria, an American doctor, John B. Ziegler, observed young Russian athletes using testosterone (Kremenik, Onodera, Nagao, Yuzuki, & Yonetani, 2006). He went home and produced a synthetic drug, based on testosterone. The drug, Dianabol, became a great success. In the 1960s, one could see bodybuilders wearing t-shirts saying: DIANABOL, BREAKFAST OF CHAMPIONS. To this end, drug use in a bodybuilding context and sport doping shared a common pre-history. As suggested by Hunt, Dimeo, Hemme, and Mueller (2014), this history can also be placed within a framework of the Cold War and the different approaches to doping found during this time in, for example, East Germany and the USA.

According to Rosen (2008), the epicenter of steroid use was to be found among weightlifters in the mythical *New York Barbell Club* (see also Fair, 1999). Steroid use spread rapidly to other sports as well as within the context of gym and fitness culture. In 1957, however, the American Medical Association raised concerns about amphetamine use in various sports. According to Dimeo (2007), the anti-doping movement was born during the mid-1950s, a movement that developed into the World Anti-Doping Agency (WADA), which today works to protect athletes' health and ensure fair play by detecting evidence of doping (Gleaves & Hunt, 2015). The long-fought war against drugs thus began, although stigmatization processes associated with drug use were quite rudimentary at the outset.

Dimeo (2007) describes this particular time in the doping history as follows:

> But we can say that there was radical change that occurred with the rise in anti-doping in the early 1960s, as campaigners collected their efforts, constructed a language to support these efforts, and developed the scientific, bureaucratic and legalistic mechanisms. This is a process that has been ignored in the historiography of sport and of medicine. (p. 6)

What Dimeo aims for, and what this section has hopefully contributed to, is a more nuanced understanding of the shift in which partial legitimacy for doping turned into an official consensus that doping (in sport) was wrong and morally dubious (see also Dimeo & Møller, 2018). As shown, the first historical phase of PIED use in the context of gym and fitness culture can be situated in parallel with and occurred in 'alliance' with modern society and sport. This period, which roughly stretches from the turn of the century to the 1960s, was characterized by optimism, scientific exploration, modernity, and a naïve understanding of the role of doping in both bodybuilding and sport.

The Sculpted and Doped Body

One central melting pot in the development of bodybuilding as well as gym and fitness culture is found on the US west coast. In the late 1930s and 1940s, a stretch of beach in Santa Monica, *Muscle Beach*, became a defining location for bodybuilding culture and lifestyles (Locks & Richardson, 2012). Here, the beachfront soon became a public space where, in the 1950s, enthusiasts could gaze at the body of icons such as Steve Reeves and others. Reeves was known for his exceptional muscular definition and aesthetic appeal. The idealizations that made Reeves famous would gradually come to change, however. In the early 1960s, when Muscle Beach was 'moved' down the coast to what was thought to be a better location, Venice Beach, a starting point for cultural transformation was initiated.

> First, bodybuilders started to appear much more defined because of the introduction of diuretics that rid the body of excess water fluid, revealing far greater levels of muscularity and definition. Second, if one looks at body-building magazines from this era, the physiques on display quite abruptly changed with an even greater impetus on mass than been seen before. [...] The reason for this change was partly due to more effective exercise and better diet, but significantly to the emergence of anabolic steroids, a factor that irreparably cut off the sport from its classical routs and would function as the primary armature of a new American Classicism which made Reeves only a nostalgic ideal. (Locks & Richardson, 2012, p. 11)

In the 1970s, gym culture and the culture of bodybuilding blossomed. From being perceived as a more or less purposeless masculine, homosocial, and subcultural preoccupation, bodybuilding was reborn, and the famous Gold's Gym in Venice Beach gradually developed from a small gym into a global franchise and cultural melting pot for bodybuilding. One driving force in this development was the documentary movie *Pumping Iron* (Gaines & Butler, 1974), in which bodybuilding icons such as Arnold Schwarzenegger, Lou Ferrigno, Franco Columbu, and Frank Zane were followed while preparing for the 1975 Mr. Olympia and Mr. Universe competitions.

Schwarzenegger was born in Thal in Austria, and in Europe during this period of time, the focus in bodybuilding was almost totally on size and mass. Upon moving to the USA, where the ideal tended toward vascularity and definition, Schwarzenegger managed to triumph on the bodybuilding scene through his ability to combine European size with American vascularity, and by doing so, he also revolutionized professional bodybuilding (Locks & Richardson, 2012). Schwarzenegger's increasing popularity and visibility gave him an international career in the film industry and later also brought him to the parlors of American politics, when he married into the Kennedy family and became the governor of California.

In the wake of Schwarzenegger's success, working out and building muscles became more or less the norm in the USA as well as elsewhere—at least among men. The health club industry also developed as part of a larger health movement, and many companies at this time were, for example, keen on providing facilities and opportunities for physical exercise to reduce the risk of heart attack and other coronary diseases among their employees (McKenzie, 2013). The body of Schwarzenegger functioned as a nexus in this development. He embodied the American dream, an ethos according to which anything is possible as long as you put your mind to it. But while Schwarzenegger did contribute greatly to making weightlifting a more common form of exercise for those who would not normally frequent a gym, he also helped make bodybuilding more extreme and subcultural as regards bodily development, size, and vascularity.

Taking bodily perfection ideals to the extreme of 'freakish' shock value, Schwarzenegger and bodybuilding in the 1970s were also entering into a new era marked by steroids. Although experimental use of synthesized testosterone occurred at various gyms on the US west coast even earlier, in the 1950s (Yesalis & Bahrke, 2007), during this later period new types of drugs were developed into customized products with far fewer and milder side effects. Thus, whereas use of PIEDs in the context of sport at this time was met with strong condemnation and preventative measures, it was largely seen as unproblematic among bodybuilders and in gym and fitness culture. In a recent interview clip on YouTube, Schwarzenegger himself talks about steroids and bodybuilding in the 1970s:

> One of the most common questions I always get is, you know, did we take steroids, because now of course drugs are such a big issue in sports. And the answer is yes. It was just in the beginning stage because bodybuilders at those days just experimented with it. But it was not illegal. It was like we talked about it very openly. I mean anyone that was asked, 'do you take steroids?', and you, 'Yeah, I take three dianabol a day' or someone else would say 'I take this, this and that.' I was not an illegal thing. (https://www.youtube.com/watch?v=uCUHjCwq_3Y)

In his revealing second autobiography *Total Recall: My Unbelievably True Life Story* (2012), Schwarzenegger and co-author Petre further develop this position, stating that there are few regrets, because this (the use of steroids) was something that came on the market and occurred under medical supervision.

The 1970s was a time of experimentation, and the legislation banning (fitness) doping was still on a very rudimentary level. For example, using steroids outside the sphere of organized sport was not only legal in most countries, but also somewhat accepted internationally, not the least in a bodybuilding context. Thus, this development and perspective on PIEDs need to be understood, first, in relation to the specificity of the time in focus and the liberal approach to experimentation in drug taking in general, prominent in the 1960s and 1970s. Second, as touched on by Schwarzenegger, we can talk about a 'pharmacological revolution' in which pharmaceutical companies increasingly began searching for and developing more potent and less toxic drugs, which could alter the biochemical, physiological, and psychological functions of the body (Verroken, 2006). Not surprisingly, bodybuilders, as well as athletes in competitive sports, saw great possibilities to utilize these chemical agents to help them push or exceed their limits, the aim being to create something new and transgress their physicality.

Female Bodybuilders—Crossing the Boundaries

Although weightlifting and bodybuilding had occurred earlier, female bodybuilding was mainly introduced in the late 1970s (Fair, 1999). Initially, there were only a few women lifting weights, and those who did enter competitions that were more like beauty contests than bodybuilding events (Klein, 1993). In this process, the male ideologues controlling bodybuilding did not encourage women to become bodybuilders. Increasingly, however, during the 1980s and 1990s, highly muscular and defined female bodies gained recognition within bodybuilding and to some extent in the public discourse. They were getting access and gradually even acceptance in the more respected circuits and gyms, and competitors such as Debbie Muggli, Lenda Murray, Iris Kyle, and Bev Francis could be seen posing with their huge and highly muscular bodies. The film *Pumping Iron II* (1985)—in which four female bodybuilders are followed while preparing for the Caesar's Palace World Cup Championship—can also be understood as part of this breakthrough.

Women thus successively entered into the subculture of male bodybuilding, signaling the start of a transformation of the whole idea of physical culture and, consequently, broadening bodybuilding as a gendered practice (Andreasson & Johansson, 2014b). Interestingly, this development paralleled a growing interest among researchers in body and gender studies, in general, and the development of feminist perspectives and theory, in particular. Scholars such as Judith Butler (1990, 1993) and Donna Haraway (1990), among others, fueled the intellectual discussion and problematization of gender and gendered bodies through their work. People began talking about stretching/exceeding the limits of the human body in different ways and about 'doing gender.' In the 1990s, scholars also turned their attention to female bodybuilders, as they were thought to represent something unique, something subversive, transgressional, and a vital challenge to hegemonic masculinity (Connell, 1995; Connell & Messerschmidt, 2005). The imagery of female bodybuilding was, however, not unambiguous.

Despite increased empowerment, the prominent theme of female bodybuilders' experience is one of contradiction, often leading to attempts to 'balance' popular notions of femininity and muscularity. Critical feminists, postmodernists, and sport sociologists describe how female bodybuilders balance contradictory demands of muscular development versus expectations of normative femininity. These include regulating muscular size to avoid being labeled as 'too big,' 'mannish,' or lesbian (...) using body technologies such as breast enlargements, plastic surgeries, and feminizing hairstyles, outfits, and accessories to counteract 'masculinizing' effects of steroid use or loss of breast tissue. (McGrath & Chananie-Hill, 2009, p. 237)

Punitive sanctions of and an explicit ideology surrounding women who were thought to violate normative gender configurations in society, used to establish boundaries around women's behavior, echo through the cultural history of gym and fitness culture. In the public discourse, female bodybuilding has often been considered a threat to the 'natural' gender order, and discussions about female bodybuilders, and female athletes in general, have tended to focus on boundaries between male/female, natural/unnatural, and on potential gender transgression with or without the use of PIEDs. To this end, female bodybuilders have historically found themselves trapped in conflicting discourses that pit sexual difference against the ethic of a universal, transcendent, and undifferentiated body culture (Lindsay, 1996; Richardsson, 2008; Roussel, Monaghan, Javerlhiac, & Yondre, 2010). Wesely (2001) also argued that PIED use and other body technologies should be viewed as representing a continuum between 'natural' and 'unnatural' bodies, emphasizing that the gender line between men and women is negotiable and changes over time and across contexts. In a similar vein, the status of the huge muscular body has changed over the period in focus here, and although gendered understandings of PIED use have prevailed to some extent, the rise of female bodybuilding as a phenomenon has signaled a movement toward gym and fitness as a mass leisure activity. At the same time, frequent reports of PIED use and the obsessional traits of bodybuilders have served as a counterweight to this development (Bunsell, 2013).

In conclusion, during the second historical phase, stretching from the 1970s into the early 1990s, gym and fitness culture broadened with regard to gender, among other things. During the golden age of bodybuilding, which came in the wake of Schwarzenegger's rampage, women gradually (and to some extent) became integrated into the previously nearly compulsory male culture and ideology. Highly muscular female and male bodies, achieved using PIEDs, became a topic of discussion not only in bodybuilding circuits, but also in the public discourse and within academia. Further, legal in most countries, steroid use was more or less seen as part of the competitive culture of bodybuilding—a perspective that, at this time, differed greatly from perspectives on doping in the context of organized sport. Entering the 1990s, however, new winds were blowing.

Confessions and Crises in Bodybuilding

At the end of the 1980s and beginning of the 1990s, bodybuilding gradually earned a bad reputation, thus entering into the *third phase* of the historical development of gym and fitness culture, in general, and fitness doping practices, in particular. Klein's (1993) now classical study on competitive bodybuilders on the American west coast deals with this process and discusses it in terms of a change in the public perspective as well as in subcultural understandings of the self within bodybuilding. Viewing themselves as nutritional and kinesiological experts, the bodybuilders of the 1980s in Klein's study are positioned at the top of the food chain in a developing culture of vanity that celebrated muscles, vitality, sexuality, control, health, and prowess. As proponents of this healthy lifestyle and culture (which included drug-using practices), Klein's bodybuilders could offer their services and counsel and train others in the art of bodybuilding, for a fee. Ironically, and in direct contrast to public declarations of fitness and health, the previously acceptance PIED use among bodybuilders began getting bad publicity. The growth of gym and fitness culture and increasing popularity of muscle-building practices were, thus, paralleled by the recognition and 'construction' of a darker side of bodybuilding (Luciano, 2001). Psychiatrists began describing a new category of young patients, obsessively preoccupied with their bodies and muscularity. In 1988, the world was also shocked by the news that sprinter Ben Johnson had used steroids. This awareness of the widespread use of drugs by athletes, but also by ordinary young men, changed things. Drugs became associated with shame and losing one's reputation as a sports(wo)man.

Consequently, through this process as well as various self-confessions, such as *Muscle: Confessions of an Unlikely Bodybuilder* (1991) by Sam Fussell, the bodybuilding subculture was thoroughly reviewed and scrutinized. Sam Fussell, the son of two university English professors, started bodybuilding at the age of 26. In September 1984, Fussell read Arnold Schwarzenegger's autobiography, *The Education of a Bodybuilder*, and decided to get involved in bodybuilding. He soon felt good, and he admired the simplicity and discipline of bodybuilding. Having felt great anxiety before, he now felt relaxed and enjoyed the routines and the hard training schedules. Soon, his body longed for the pump and the pain. Upon arriving in California and at Gold's gym, he also began using steroids. One man at the gym, Vinnie, introduced him to the drugs. Fussell writes: 'That very day, Vinnie began my education as a bodybuilder and instructed me on the merits of performance-enhancing drugs' (p. 118). He soon discovered that his heroes and the best bodybuilders ever were all on steroids. By the late 1980s, steroid use had exploded in the USA. Fussell was well educated and soon he was using a wide variety of drugs in his training. Although he was aware of the possible side effects, he also began to use the needle.

> And there were other little problems from the drugs, the sheet said, problems like premature baldness, lowered sperm count, increased body hair, rectal bleeding, dizzy spells, thyroid and liver and kidney malfunction, gallstones, cancer, gastrointestinal upset, hepatitis, raised levels of aggression /…/. (p. 121)

Fussell told himself that he was making a bargain with the devil, in exchange for transcending his body and creating something extraordinary. Although his training gave results, he started to feel alienated from himself, his parents and society. Looking at himself in the mirror, he was no longer sure that bodybuilding was the right way to go. Gradually, he discovered that he had to leave the sport and life of bodybuilding and to continue his life, following another path. Leaving the bodybuilding lifestyle was not easy, however.

Despite all I knew, leaving iron wasn't that simple, of course. No iron veteran after all, just walks away. Without the buttresses and corbels, the brackets and bolstering devices of muscles, bodybuilders feel they'd collapse quicker than a house of cards. It's no wonder the rate of recidivism is astronomically high, and all my gym friends assumed that I'd be no exception. (p. 250)

In June 2014, the journalist Michael J. Joyner located Sam Fussell and interviewed him. Writing his self-revealing and critical book was very much an attempt at self-exile from bodybuilding. Fussell understood that he would no longer be welcomed by his old friends or at the gym. After releasing the book, he was constantly on tour, talking about it and his life as a former bodybuilder. He explains:

Initially, when my book came out 1991, I did talk show after talk show and I was pitted against bodybuilders who lied through their teeth, claiming the best bodybuilders in the world never took steroids, etc. I understood why they lied: they'd say anything to protect that which they loved. /…/PED's have been such a given and used by 100% of the top competitors in the world that it becomes a kind of club. Everyone in the club knows. Everyone in the clubs knows that the first rule of the Fight Club is there is no Fight Club. (Joyner, 2014)

Fussell continued to reveal more about the drugs in the interview. Using steroids, he could train several times a day, and he could also have several orgasms each night with his girlfriend. Steroids were like amphetamines for him, he said. However, as he understood it, openly talking about this, and drug use in bodybuilding in general, was however not appreciated by the bodybuilding community. Consequently, his strategy of distancing himself from and exiting the world of bodybuilding and steroids was also 'supported' by former bodybuilding friends. Today, Fussell has left the culture of bodybuilding and works as a hunting guide in Montana.

Fussell's book helped create ripples on the water, presenting a strong critique of American machismo. In a similar vein, Klein's (1993) study on American west coast bodybuilders helped reveal a hyper-masculine sub-culture marked by homophobia and misogyny, but paradoxically also by homosexual hustling. At this time, building muscle by using steroids was largely understood as a means to compensate for vulnerable, insecure masculinity, among other things. By building a bodily fortress, flaws and insecurities were thought to be disguised (see also Chapter 7). Consequently, in the third historical phase of fitness doping, we find complex movements in which the doped bodybuilding masculinity and bodybuilding culture are questioned, at the same time as women continue to gradually enter and gain a position in this culture. The issue of health becomes paramount, as do discussions on the side effects of PIED use observed among men and women.

The Fitness Revolution—Cleaning Up the Mess

In the late 1990s and especially when moving forward to the first two decades of the twenty-first century, we see an explosion of fitness franchises and more and more people being drawn into fitness. Entering the *fourth phase* of the historical development of gym culture and fitness doping, the subculture of bodybuilding is gradually disconnected from the more general trend of fitness gyms and from conceiving of the gym as a place for everyone, and a mass leisure activity with strong health and sound lifestyle connotations (Sassatelli, 2010; Smith Maguire, 2008). The effects of drug use in bodybuilding were thoroughly investigated, and more controls were made at gyms. A Danish study showed, for example, that fitness franchises, such as SATS and Fitness World, used drug tests to keep up a good reputation and to remove bodybuilders from their gyms (Mogensen, 2011). Sassatelli (2010) describes this process of cultural relocation in the following way:

> As is apparent, today the term "gym" is associated with that of "fitness" and even increasingly replaced by neologisms lite "fitness centre" or "fitness club" which, as some clients and trainers claim, better convey the specific mission of this institution. To be sure, gyms reserved solely for typically masculine competitive activities—such as body building, weightlifting, boxing or the martial arts—still exist, but they are increasingly marginal with respect to the large number of premises that find a minimum common denomination in the idea of fitness. (p. 17)

The fitness revolution of the 1990s can also be seen as a reaction to the falling star of bodybuilders and an attempt to sanitize the sport. Frequent reports on drug use and anabolic steroids, combined with the obsessive features of bodybuilding, led to diminishing interest in bodybuilding. The gradual cultural separation between bodybuilding and fitness does not mean that these phenomena have become two different activities and lifestyles, however. These conceptions of exercise and lifestyle are partly disconnected from each other and partly increasingly dependent on each other.

In response to the growing fitness enterprise, in many countries there was also a struggle among certain practitioners to prevent heavy commercialization of the gym culture and the development of commercialized lifestyle concepts. In the USA, for example, the YMCA tried for a long time to keep at bay the commercial aspects of the business and to make it possible for young people to exercise for free (Miller & Fielding, 1995). Also, many bodybuilders have proven to be quite critical of the commercialization, which is thought to threaten the fundamental character or essence of the physical culture bodybuilding developed from (Andreasson & Johansson, 2014b; Monaghan, 2001, 2012). But eventually many organizations adapted to the global development, turning into regular businesses. Fitness has become the overall concept used when referring to health clubs and fitness franchises and has thereby turned into a popular movement—not one comparable to the old twentieth-century movements, often connected to national sentiments, but instead a highly individualized and personal task (Andreasson & Johansson, 2014a).

As regards female bodybuilding, which gained increasing recognition during the 1980s and early 1990s, the picture has changed since the turn of the century. On an organizational level, the governing body of bodybuilding and fitness, the *International Federation of Bodybuilding and Fitness* (IFBB), began increasingly insisting that women must maintain their 'female forms' and muscle definition. In line with this, the concept and discipline of *Women's Fitness* was introduced in 1996, paving the way for a 'less muscular and aesthetically pleasing physique' and ideal for female bodybuilders (IFBB, 2018). Later disciplines such as *Women Body-fitness* and *Women's Bikini-Fitness* were also added, further accentuating the marginalization of female bodybuilding. As a consequence, competitors who previously lost against more muscular bodybuilders have returned to the sport and won competitions.

In many ways, this development can be understood as a means by which organizers and central stakeholders in bodybuilding and fitness have aimed to adjust the sport's development, adapting it to what is considered a more traditional gender order. Of course, as the female bodybuilding bodies of the 1990s steadily grew in mass and vascularity, discussions on fitness doping followed. This development also related to central stakeholders' efforts to deal with the doping stigma in bodybuilding. The marginalization of female bodybuilding and the boosting of disciplines such as women's bikini fitness have helped make the connection between the modern gym and health paramount. We will soon return to a discussion on how these processes have impacted the fitness doping demography of the twenty-first century. Before doing so, however, we will shortly address a recent development in bodybuilding that can be understood in relation to the bad reputation of bodybuilding and the desire to reattach bodybuilding to the growth of a more general fitness trend.

Natural Bodies and Bodybuilding

The face of gym and fitness has changed, and we can talk about a globalized fitness revolution. Whereas in this process bodybuilding has often been associated with things such as steroids, vanity, and hyper-masculinity, fitness has been constructed in accordance with values such as health, youth, and beauty. Efforts to deal with the 'black-sheep' stigma and bad reputation of bodybuilding have included the development of *natural bodybuilding*.

Natural, that is drug free, bodybuilding has developed rapidly during recent decades. It has become a distinct culture, with competitions, events, promoters, and federations. The emergence of a broader movement toward natural bodybuilding can be located to the late 1980s and early 1990s (Liokaftos, 2018). This development coincides with stricter regulations on steroids in the USA. According to Liokaftos, the movement toward natural bodybuilding is also connected to a number of premature deaths of well-known bodybuilders, such as Mohammed Benaziza (1992) and Andreas Munzer (1996). Their deaths were directly linked to substance abuse in connection with competitions, and as a consequence, in the 1990s there was a growing social movement within bodybuilding promoting natural bodybuilding. This movement has been made visible through new bodybuilding media as well as the development of new organizations and organized sporting activities.

Supporters of natural bodybuilding have mobilized two discourses (Liokaftos, 2018). The first is about choice, suggesting that athletes should be able to practice and compete in the sport without feeling the need and pressure to use drugs. The second discourse is focused on the values and ethos of bodybuilding. Relying on values, such as health, character building, and fair competitions, natural bodybuilding is trying to establish an alternative to PIED use. This movement is also interconnected with the development of more general anti-doping and anti-drug organizations in society, of course, and from the 2000s onwards, we can see the consolidation and global expansion of natural bodybuilding.

To conclude, in the fourth phase of the historical development of fitness doping, strong efforts are made to 'clean up' gym and fitness culture. Health and fitness are constructed as paramount ideals and premises for weightlifting, resulting in fitness palaces for a diverse demographic of training enthusiasts. Bodybuilding remains and continues to offer new ideas about training and how to form bodies through dieting and hard work (and PIEDs). At the same time, bodybuilding is largely marginalized in this new culture of fitness and firm bodies. Although natural bodybuilding shares many of the visions of bodybuilding in general—rationalization, productivity, and the self as a project—it is also an alternative to getting involved in the riskier and more (presumably) deviant milieus of bodybuilding. Naturally, it is also possible to discern a dynamic relation between extreme bodybuilding—where drugs and PIEDs are inherent parts of the sport—and natural bodybuilding. The latter offers a way out from subcultural and drug-saturated environments and competitions. Natural bodybuilding is also more in line with the general development of fitness culture in society, and with a normalization of the sport.

A Globalized (and Virtual) Drug Market—Entering a Fifth Phase?

As touched upon throughout this chapter, PIED use has continued and can be argued to have broadened demographically, internationally, since the late 1970s (Antonopoulos & Hall, 2016; Bates & McVeigh, 2016). Previously seen almost exclusively as a problem within elite sport, the use of doping and the doping market have 'spread' to gym culture, to male body-builders, then female bodybuilders, non-elite athletes, and more recently among what is perceived to be regular gym-goers or mainstream fitness groups (Hanley Santos & Coomber, 2017; McVeigh, Bates, & Chandler, 2015). As a consequence of this historical development, the profile and market for potential users seem also to have diversified, as has the literature on the reasons for and experiences of PIED use (see, e.g., Christiansen, 2018; Christiansen, Schmidt Vinther, & Liokaftos, 2016; Kimegård & McVeigh, 2014; Sagoe et al., 2015). Not surprisingly, in line with processes of globalization of gym and fitness culture and increasing diversification of the fitness doping demography, the supply and range of available (illicit and licit) PIEDs have also widened (Coomber et al., 2015; Fincoeur, van de Ven & Mulrooney, 2015; Van Hout & Kean, 2015). This development has further been powered by the possibility to use the Internet to discuss, learn about, and deal PIEDs (a topic we will return to in Chapter 6). As suggested by van de Ven and Mulrooney (2017), however, scholars have primarily focused on how we can understand users' perspectives on con-sumption and, thus, have to some extent neglected methods and models for understanding the supply side of the fitness doping market.

Roughly, in an historical perspective, the market and distribution of fitness doping follows a route similar to the development of gym and fit-ness culture described in this chapter. In the 1980s and 1990s, the doping market often followed a social, and less commercially driven, model (van de Ven & Mulrooney, 2017). Here, dealing networks were mainly was built on well-developed relationships between sellers and buyers. Put dif-ferently, experienced users/bodybuilders often 'helped out' and supported new friends at the gym, not only supplying the drugs but also mentoring them on how to use PIEDs (Andreasson & Johansson, 2016; Monaghan,

2001, 2012). To this end, the doping market was somewhat embedded in the local and cultural spatiality of the gym and bodybuilding culture.

Since the turn of the century, however, and as a consequence of stricter anti-doping policies and regulations, this has changed. The inherent risks of encounters with the police, in some countries, have diminished the level of sociability among fitness doping suppliers. Instead, there is a growing market of online communities and possibilities, through which socioculturally embedded suppliers are being replaced with profit-driven dealers (Fincoeur et al., 2015). Thus, a new type of online market with commercially motivated suppliers is evolving (van de Ven & Mulrooney, 2017). Fully in line with neoliberal values, we now have a process of globalization through which the doping market is gradually being transformed from a socioculturally embedded to a disembedded and commercialist market, existing on an international and most often virtual and anonymous arena. Needless to say, this displacement does not only entail a great challenge for national anti-doping policies and law enforcement. It also entails the risk of increasing drug use and loss of social support and mentoring of use.

Conclusions

The first phase of the history of contemporary fitness doping derives from a pre-history of bodybuilding and can be connected to *physical culture* and the strongmen of the early twentieth century. Putting their developed bodies on display in a time of modernity, men such as Eugen Sandow and Charles Atlas presented something unique in terms of muscularity, and in doing so, they also made their way into the history books and bodybuilding hall of fame. This period of time was in many respects formative for the development of gym culture and bodybuilding, not least concerning the training techniques used to mold the bodies of men. Yet this formative phase is only a starting point.

The development within bodybuilding from the 1970s onwards— establishment of the IFBB, the stardom of Arnold Schwarzenegger and others, the rise of female bodybuilding, and the medialization of bodybuilding and fitness—can be interpreted as part of a second phase. In contrast to the pre-historical development, here we also see a development toward a global culture, accentuated by the medialization of society, and the development of a global business enterprise. Whereas within sports in general the discussion on fitness doping (read steroids) in the 1960s and 1970s led to legislation and increasingly developed control systems, body-building seemed to have created a secluded space for improving and using steroids and other substances. However, the optimism and celebration of PIEDs observed in the second phase gradually turned into a crisis and a more critical approach to bodybuilding, in general, and to the health risks associated with drug use practices, in particular. During the late 1980s and the 1990s, bodybuilding and its associated lifestyle were questioned in the public discourse—a time described in this chapter as a third phase—and in order to preserve and develop gym and fitness culture, strong attempts were made to dissociate fitness culture from bodybuilding, especially from the use of illicit substances. This can be interpreted as a kind of 'civilizing process,' where the whole gym and fitness culture gradually changed its appearance and became something quite new and different from the sub-cultural forms of bodybuilding we saw in the 1970s in the USA, Sweden, and other countries. This fourth phase, which has been referred to as the *Fitness Revolution*, is largely connected to the changed spatiality of the gym, the development of new disciplines in the more competitive parts of the culture, and a general diversification of the gym demography. Gym culture transformed into a fitness enterprise in which drug use practices and bodybuilding were exiled to a certain extent.

What we see today, however, may be the initiation of a *fifth phase* in this historical development. Increasingly, we have discussions on the effectiveness of the control systems created and on how to develop more holistic approaches to drug use in sports (Hanstad & Waddington, 2009; Waddington & Smith, 2009). There are also critical discussions on the stigmatization of, for example, *Human Growth Hormones* (HGH). López (2012) argues that there is a lack of evidence for the deleterious and fatal side effects of HGH. Furthermore, López claims that the alarming reports on the health dangers associated with HGH were popularized and grad-ually came to be naturalized by the media. Through repetition and a lack of confrontation with critical investigations, HGH came to be defined as detrimental to athletes' health. Critics of the anti-doping position are slowly gaining ground. Gleaves (2010) contends that harmless PIEDs may be manufactured in the future. This development can of course also be situated in relation to the medicalization of society, which is a societal process characterized by a rationality, common within modern medicine, according to which pharmaceuticals provide quick and easy solutions to a variety of physical problems, and as such benefitting from them is logical. In order to continue the anti-doping work, there will probably be a need to elaborate other types of arguments and values, more connected, for example, to the intrinsic values of sport and the ethical ideals of natural bodybuilding.

Also, as Thualagant (2012) points out, PIED use can paradoxically be seen as a way to achieve social integration. In a society where performance culture and neoliberal ideals concerning successful bodies are encouraged, drugs become a means of reaching one's goals. By optimizing one's human and bodily capital—through the use of PIEDs—the individual can fulfill the dream of the perfect body (Markula, 2001). However, as the ideals and image of the perfect body gradually become more impossible to reach within the limits of 'natural bodybuilding,' the temptations to use other, and often illegal, means to reach one's goals will grow.

References

Al-Falasi, O., Al-Dahmani, K., & Al-Eisaei, K. (2008). Knowledge, attitude and practice of anabolic steroids use among gym users in Al-Ain District, United Arab Emirates. *The Open Sports Medicine Journal, 9*(2), 75–81.

Allahverdipour, H., Jalilian, F., & Shaghaghi, A. (2012). Vulnerability and the intention to anabolic steroids use among Iranian gym users: An application of the theory of planned behavior. *Substance Use and Misuse, 47,* 309–312.

Andreasson, J., & Johansson, T. (2014a). The fitness revolution: Historical transformations in the global gym and fitness culture. *Sport Science Review, XXIII*(3–4), 91–112.

Andreasson, J., & Johansson, T. (2014b). *The global gym: Gender, health and pedagogies.* Basingstoke, UK: Palgrave Macmillan.

Andreasson, J., & Johansson, T. (2016). Online doping: The new self-help culture of ethnopharmacology. *Sport in Society: Cultures, Media, Politics, Commerce, 19*(7), 957–972.

Antonopoulos, G. A., & Hall, A. (2016). 'Gain with no pain': Anabolic-androgenic steroids trafficking in the UK. *European Journal of Criminology, 13*(6), 696–713. https://doi.org/10.1177/1477370816633261.

Bates, G., & McVeigh, J. (2016). *Image and performance enhancing drugs: 2015 survey results.* Liverpool: Liverpool John Moores University.

Budd, M. A. (1997). *The sculpture machine: Physical culture and body politics in the age of empire.* London: Macmillan Press.

Bunsell, T. (2013). *Strong and hard women: An ethnography of female bodybuilding.* London: Routledge.

Butler, J. (1990). *Gender trouble: Feminism and the subversion of identity.* London: Routledge.

Butler, J. (1993). *Bodies that matter: On the discursive limits of "sex".* London: Routledge.

Christiansen, A. V. (2018). Motionsdoping. Styrketræning, identitet og kultur [Recreational doping. Strength training, identity and culture]. Aarhus, Denmark: Aarhus Universitetsforlag.

Christiansen, A. V., Schmidt Vinther, A., & Liokaftos, D. (2016). Outline of a typology of men's use of anabolic androgenic steroids in fitness and strength training environments. *Drugs: Education, Prevention and Policy, 24*(3), 295–305. http://doi.org/10.1080/09687637.2016.1231173

Connell, R. W. (1995). *Masculinities.* Cambridge, MA: Polity Press.

Connell, R. W., & Messerschmidt, J. W. (2005). Hegemonic masculinity: Rethinking the concept. *Gender & Society, 19,* 829–859.

Connolly, J. (2015). Civilising processes and doping in professional cycling. *Current Sociology, 63*(7), 1037–1057.

Coomber, R., Pavlidis, A., Santos, G. H., Wilde, M., Schmidt, W., & Redshaw, C. (2015). The supply of steroids and other performance and image enhancing drugs (PIEDs) in one English city: Fakes, counterfeits, supplier trust, common beliefs and access. *Performance Enhancement and Health, 3*(3–4), 135–144. https://doi.org/10.1016/j.peh.2015.10.004.

Dimeo, P. (2007). *A history of drug use in sport 1876–1976: Beyond good and evil.* London: Routledge.

Dimeo, P., & Hunt, T. M. (2011). The doping of athletes in the former East Germany: A critical assessment of comparison with Nazi medical experiments. *International Review for Sociology of Sport, 47*(5), 581–593.

Dimeo, P., & Møller, V. (2018). *The anti-doping crisis in sport: Causes, consequences, solutions.* London: Routledge.

Evans-Brown, M., McVeigh, J., Perkins, C., & Bellis, M. A. (2012). *Human enhancement drugs: The emerging challenges to public health.* Liverpool: North West Public Health Observatory.

Fair, J. D. (1999). *Muscletown USA: Bob Hoffman and the manly culture of York Barbell.* University Park: The Pennsylvania State University Press.

Fincoeur, B., van de Ven, K., & Mulrooney, K. (2015). The symbiotic evolution of anti-doping and supply chains of doping substances: How criminal networks may benefit from anti-doping policy. *Trends in Organized Crime, 18*(3), 229–250. https://doi.org/10.1007/s12117-014-9235-7.

Fussell, S. (1991). *Muscle: Confessions of an unlikely bodybuilder.* London: Scribners.

Gaines, C., & Butler, G. (1974). *Pumping iron: The art and sport of bodybuilding.* London: Sphere Books.

Gleaves, J. (2010). No harm, no foul? Justifying bans on safe performance-enhancing drugs. *Sport, Ethics and Philosophy, 4*(3), 269–283.

Gleaves, J., & Hunt, T. (Eds.). (2015). *A global history of doping in sport: Drugs, policy, and politics.* London: Routledge.

Hanley Santos, G., & Coomber, R. (2017). The risk environment of anabolic—Androgenic steroid users in the UK: Examining motivations, practices and accounts of use. *International Journal of Drug Policy, 40,* 35–43. https://doi.org/10.1016/j.drugpo.2016.11.005.

Hanstad, D.-V., & Waddington, I. (2009). Sport, health and drugs: A critical re-examination of some key issues and problems. *Perspectives in Public Health, 129*(4), 174–182.

Haraway, D. (1990). A manifesto for cyborgs: Science, technology and socialist feminism in the 1980's. In Nicholson, L. J. (Ed.), *Feminism/postmodernism.* London: Routledge.

Hoff, D. (2013). Dopning utanför idrotten – individualisering och muskulösa skönhetsideal. En studie av dopning i grundskola, gymnasium och på gym i Kalmar kommun. *Scandinavian Sport Studies Forum, 4,* 1–24.

Holt, I. G., Iouletta, E.-M., & Sönksen, P. H. (2009). The history of doping and growth hormone abuse in sport. *Growth Hormone & IGF Research, 19*(4), 320–326.

Hunt, T., Dimeo, P., Hemme, F., & Mueller, A. (2014). The health risks of doping during the cold war: A comparative analysis of the two sides of the Iron Curtain. *The International Journal of the History of Sport, 31*(17), 2230–2244.

IFBB. (2018). *Our disciplines.* Retrieved 3 October 2018 https://ifbb.com/our-disciplines/.

Joyner, M. J. (2014). *Sam Fussell: An interview with the author of muscle.* Human limits, a blogg by Joyner, M.

Kimegård, A. (2015). A qualitative study of anabolic steroid use amongst gym users in the United Kingdom: Motives, beliefs and experiences. *Journal of Substance Use, 20*(4), 288–294.

Kimegård, A., & McVeigh, J. (2014). Variability and dilemmas in harm reduction for anabolic steroid users in the UK: A multi-area interview study. *Harm Reduction Journal, 11*(1), 1–13. https://doi.org/10.1186/1477-7517-11-19.

Klein, A. (1993). *Little big men: Bodybuilding, subculture and gender construction.* New York: State University of New York Press.

Kremenik, M., Onodera, S., Nagao, M., Yuzuki, O., & Yonetani, S. (2006). A historical timeline of doping in the Olympics (Part 1 1896–1968). *Kawasaki Journal of Medical Welfare, 12*(1), 19–28.

Lindsay, C. (1996). Bodybuilding: A postmodern freak show. In R. G. Thomson (Ed.), *Freakery: Cultural spectacles of the extraordinary body.* New York: New York University Press.

Liokaftos, D. (2018). Natural bodybuilding: An account of its emergence and development as competition sport. *International Review for the Sociology of Sport.* https://doi.org/10.1177/1012690217751439.

Locks, A., & Richardson, N. (2012). *Critical readings in bodybuilding.* London: Routledge.

López, B. (2012). Creating fear: The social construction of human Growth Hormone as a dangerous drug. *International Review for the Sociology of Sports, 48*(2), 220–237.

Luciano, L. (2001). *Looking good: Male body image in modern America.* New York: Hill and Wang.

Markula, P. (2001). Beyond the perfect body: Women's body image distortion in fitness magazine discourse. *Journal of Sport & Social Issues, 25*(2), 158–179.

McGrath, S., & Chananie-Hill, R. (2009). 'Big Freaky-Looking Women': Normalizing gender transgression through bodybuilding. *Sociology of Sport Journal, 26*, 235–254.

McKenzie, S. (2013). *Getting physical: The rise of fitness culture in America.* Lawrence: University Press of Kansas.

McVeigh, J., Bates, G., & Chandler, M. (2015). *Steroids and image enhancing drugs—2014 survey results.* Retrieved from Liverpool: http://www.ipedinfo.co.uk/resources/downloads/SIEDs%20Survey%20report%202014%20FINAL.pdf.

Miller, L. K., & Fielding, L. W. (1995). The battle between the for-profit health club and the 'commercial' YMCA. *Journal of Sport and Social Issues, 19*(1), 76–107.

Mogensen, K. (2011). *Body Punk. En afhandling om mandlige kropsbyggere og kroppens betydninger i lyset av antidoping kampagner* [Body punk: A thesis on male bodybuilders and the meanings of the body in the light of anti-doping campaigns]. Roskilde: Roskilde Universitetscenter.

Monaghan, L. (2001). *Bodybuilding, drugs and risk: Health, risk and society.* New York: Routledge.

Monaghan, L. F. (2012). Accounting for illicit steroid use: Bodybuilders' justifications. In A. Locks, & N. Richardson (Ed.), *Critical readings in bodybuilding.* New York: Routledge.

Petrocelli, M., Oberweis, T., & Petrocelli, J. (2008). Getting huge, getting ripped: A qualitative exploration of recreational steroid use. *Journal of Drug Issues, 2008*(Fall), 1187–1206.

Pineau, T., Schopfer, A., Grossrieder, L., Broséus, J., Esseiva, P., & Rossy, Q. (2016). The study of doping market: How to produce intelligence from internet forums. *Forensic Science International, 268*(2016), 103–115.

Pope, H. G., Kanayama, G., Athey, A., Ryan, E., Hudson, J. I., & Baggish, A. (2014). The lifetime prevalence of anabolic-androgenic steroid use and dependence in Americans: Current best estimates. *The American Journal on Addictions, 23*(4), 371–377.

Richardson, N. (2008). Flex-rated! Female bodybuilding: Feminist resistance or erotic spectacle? *Journal of Gender Studies, 17*(4), 289–301.

Rosen, D. M. (2008). *A history of performance enhancement in sports from the nineteenth century to today.* Westport: Praeger.

Roussel, P., Monaghan, L., Javerlhiac, S., & Yondre, F. (2010). The metamorphosis of female bodybuilders: Judging a paroxysmal body? *International Review for the Sociology of Sport, 45*(1), 103–109.

Sagoe, D., McVeigh, J., Bjørnebekk, A., Essilfie, M. S., Andreassen, C. S., & Pallesen, S. (2015). Polypharmacy among anabolic-androgenic steroid users: A descriptive metasynthesis. *Substance Abuse: Treatment, Prevention, and Policy, 10*(1). http://doi.org/10.1186/s13011-015-0006-5.

Santos, A. M., Da Rocha, M. S. P., & Da Silva, M. F. (2011). Illicit use and abuse of anabolic-androgenic steroids among Brazilian bodybuilders. *Substance Use and Misuse, 46,* 742–748.

Sassatelli, R. (2010). *Fitness culture: Gyms and the commercialisation of discipline and fun.* Hampshire: Palgrave Macmillan.

Schwarzenegger, A., & Petre, P. (2012). *Total recall: My unbelievably true life story.* New York, NY: Simon & Schuster.

Smith Maguire, J. (2008). *Fit for consumption: Sociology and the business of fitness.* London and New York: Routledge.

Thualagant, N. (2012). The conceptualization of fitness doping and its limitations. *Sport in Society: Cultures, Commerce, Media, Politics, 15*(3), 409–419.

Van de Ven, K., & Mulrooney, K. (2017). Social suppliers: Exploring the cultural contours of the performance and image enhancing drug (PIED) market among bodybuilders in the Netherlands and Belgium. *International Journal of Drug Policy, 40,* 6–15. https://doi.org/10.1016/j.drugpo.2016.07.009.

Van Hout, M. C., & Kean, J. (2015). An exploratory study of image and performance enhancement drug use in a male British South Asian community. *International Journal of Drug Policy, 26*(9), 860–867. https://doi.org/10.1016/j.drugpo.2015.03.002.

Verroken, M. (2006). Drug use and abuse in sport. In D. R. Mottram (Ed.), *Drugs in sport* (4th ed., pp. 29–63). London and New York: Routledge.

Vertinsky, P. (1999). Making and marking gender: Bodybuilding and the medicalization of the body from one century's end to another. *Culture, Sport, Society, 2*(1), 1–24.

Waddington, I., & Smith, A. (2009). *An introduction to drugs in sport: Addicted to winning?.* New York: Routledge.

Wesely, J. K. (2001). Negotiating gender: Bodybuilding and the natural/unnatural continuum. *Sociology of Sport Journal, 18*(2), 162–180.

Yesalis, C., & Bahrke, M. (2007). Anabolic steroid and stimulant use in North American sport between 1850 and 1980. In P. Dimeo (Ed.), *Drugs, alcohol and sport.* New York: Routledge.

3

Glocal Fitness Doping

Introduction

In 2010, the American bodybuilding icon Jay Cutler was invited to guest pose at an annual bodybuilding competition in Sweden called the Lucia Trophy as part of the Fitness Festival—the largest fitness fair and expo in Northern Europe. The competition organizers had marketed heavily on Cutler's presence, aiming to attract large numbers of visitors. Instead of flexing muscles, however, a video was played on a big screen in which Cutler, from his home in the USA, said the following to the Swedish audience:

> This is Jay Cutler from Las Vegas. I understand you have a packed house at the Fitness Festival in Gothenburg today. Let me tell you this; I would have loved to be there and guest pose for you. But; as you know, this week Toney Freeman was taken by the police in Sweden and brought in for questioning. I have talked to Toney. He says that this happened just because

---

This chapter builds upon an article that was published in *Performance Enhancement and Health* and authored by Jesper Andreasson and April Henning at the University of Stirling, UK.

J. Andreasson and T. Johansson, *Fitness Doping*,
https://doi.org/10.1007/978-3-030-22105-8_3

he is a professional bodybuilder. /.../ Having seen how this damaged Toney Freeman via the Internet, I simply could not risk to face the same. So, based on advice given to me here in the US, I decided that I could not come to Sweden this time. (Jay Cutler)

Following the video, the crowd booed and whistled their disappointment, and the conferencier concluded over the speakers that the anti-doping work done by Swedish police should be understood as 'nothing other than an attack on the sport of bodybuilding' (observational note). As the situation above illustrates, understandings and use of doping in the gym and bodybuilding context can vary by country. Likewise, anti-doping legislation, preventative work, and how each are understood by practitioners and potential users vary as well. In the above situation, the different ways of approaching and understanding doping in terms of policy, practice, and prevention seem to intersect and implode on one occasion—at a fitness fair in a small country in northern Europe.

In this chapter, we will discuss and analyze how fitness doping can be understood in relation to, and how it is affected by, different national and local contexts. Because the two countries represent different forms of welfare state regimes, we will focus on fitness doping in the USA and Sweden. Our analysis will be sociologically informed and structured in relation to three central aspects of fitness doping: policy, practice, and prevention (cf. Hall & Jefferson, 1976). We are interested in questions such as: How has legislation on the use of doping developed over time? How is fitness doping discussed by users in the selected countries? We will also pay attention to the kinds of preventative work that are (or are not) being conducted. The idea is to present a comparative analysis of two rather different national approaches to fitness doping, situated within the context of a globalized, Western gym and fitness culture.

The Hegemony and Limitations of WADA

Historically, anti-doping efforts have focused on the detection and deterrence of doping in formally governed competitions in (elite) sports contexts (European Commission, 2014). Researchers have studied the ways in which WADA has operated in its effort to develop effective anti-doping policies and combat doping in sport on a global scale. WADA introduced an international World Anti-Doping Code to which all countries and international sport organizations would be expected to subscribe (Hanstad & Houlihan, 2015). The role of WADA and its affiliated National Anti-Doping Organizations (NADOs) was solidified when stakeholders quickly signed onto the World Anti-Doping Code and when governments were equally quick to ratify the 2007 UNESCO Convention Against Doping in Sport, which bound governments to support implementation of the WADA Code (Hanstad & Houlihan, 2015). In the wake of these developments, concern over doping outside the formally governed sports context—WADA's jurisdiction—also emerged (European Commission, 2014).

As touched on in Chapter 2, since the late 1990s and especially during the first two decades of the twenty-first century, there has been an explosion of fitness franchises, drawing more people into fitness activities (Andreasson & Johansson, 2014; Sassatelli, 2010). Paradoxically, at the same time cultural fitness trends have gained momentum, the resulting emphasis on the body and its appearance has contributed to persistent doping problems (Christiansen, 2018; Liokaftos, 2012; McGrath & Chananie-Hill, 2009). Policymakers' efforts to legislate against doping and public health organizations' efforts to promote drug-free physical activities in these contexts have further contributed to marginalizing drug use practices in the public discourse (see, e.g., Andreasson & Johansson, 2016; Monaghan, 2001). Among other things, this has boosted the emergence of new globalized arenas for fitness doping through social media and different Internet forums, for example. This has been discussed in several studies, which, in different ways, have raised the question of how online communication can contribute to users' awareness and initiation into doping in a context not bound by national laws, policies, and prevention strategies (see Andreasson, 2015; Monaghan, 2012; Smith & Stewart, 2012). We will return to this discussion in Chapter 6.

The European Commission brought together a group of experts in 2011 to further investigate the landscape of fitness doping. The report showed, among other things, that in the 28 EU member states, as many as 17 national coordinators for anti-doping could not identify or name any 'good' prevention practices. Whereas Austria, for example, presented only general advice on how to pursue prevention in the field of doping by naming YouTube videos, countries such as Denmark have regularly conducted doping controls in fitness clubs. Overall, few examples of evaluated doping prevention programs were noted (European Commission, 2014, p. 64). The report further emphasized that representation of the Nordic countries was significant in terms of developed programs, and that these programs were most often community-based and focused on educating personal trainers, gym owners, and fitness athletes through various anti-doping campaigns.

Fitness Doping in the USA and Sweden

As regards the situation in the USA and Sweden, which is in focus for this chapter, a few comments can be made. In the USA, decisions to regulate anabolic substances have frequently been in response to moral panics around formally governed sport and concerns over use by young athletes (Denham, 2006). The annual *Monitoring the Future* youth survey reported that lifetime steroid use dropped to 1.2% in 2017 from its high of 3.3% in 2001–2002 among 8th, 10th, and 12th grade students combined (Johnston et al., 2018). However, this same report showed a decline in perceived risk of using steroids to a record low of 49% of students seeing great risk (Johnston et al., 2018). While youth use may have been a driver for legislation, they are far from the only group to use PIEDs in the USA. A meta-analysis of the general population found that age of first anabolic use is largely (78%) after age 20, which is later than the onset of other types of drug use (Pope et al., 2014). The same study estimated that between 2.9 and 4 million Americans have used anabolic substances in their lifetimes (Pope et al., 2014).

Concerning the situation in Sweden (fitness), doping as a societal problem was recognized by the Public Health Agency in Sweden in the late 1980s (Statens Folkhälsoinstitut, 2011) and further addressed through implementation of an anti-doping act in 1992. Few surveys have been conducted looking at the extent of Swedish doping, in general, and fitness doping, in particular. But one survey study carried out at schools in a municipality in southern Sweden showed that 1% of girls and 2% of boys in elementary school and 2% of high school girls and boys reported use of banned substances (Hoff, 2013). At fitness centers, 4% of women and 5% of men reported doping use, most commonly in the 31–35 (15%) age group. We will return to the policy, practice, and prevention situations in both the USA and Sweden later in the chapter.

Welfare Regimes and Doping

In contextualizing our case studies on the situation in the USA and Sweden, the work of Danish sociologist Gøsta Esping-Andersen (1990) has been useful. Esping-Andersen developed a model that has been used when comparing different welfare regimes, predominantly in Europe and the West. The model identifies and categorizes clusters of nations that represent different political ambitions and perspectives on, for example, individual responsibility/freedom and social policies. Although the model has often been used to try to understand the relationship between the state, the capitalist market, and the individual in terms of social class and gender, it has utility here in helping us contextualize how fitness doping has been approached in terms of policy and structure within the specific contexts of the USA and Sweden. The cluster of nations that includes the USA is the *liberal welfare state regimes*, which are characterized by the twin ideologies of individual responsibility/freedom and reduced government found within neoliberal discourses. Another cluster of nations, where we find Sweden, is the *Nordic welfare states*. These are often referred to as social democratic and characterized by more general social security systems in the public sector. One key tenet is that social policy is developed to redistribute resources so as to achieve equality among citizens. Esping-Andersen also describes a third cluster of nations called the *conservative welfare state regimes*, which includes for example Germany, Belgium, and France. These are developed welfare policy regimes, but they provide less extensive economic support for the public sector than do the Nordic states.

There are limitations to Esping-Andersen's model (see Esping-Andersen, 2009). Critics have emphasized that the typology marginalizes certain countries, such as those in Central and Eastern Europe (Hearn &

Pringle, 2009; Pierson, 1998). Others have argued that the model does not sufficiently take the role of public services and gender politics into account and have attempted to develop alternative typologies (Bambra, 2004, 2007). But Esping-Andersen's model nevertheless provides a broad tool for discussing the characteristics of different welfare state models and the impact they may have, in this case, on how fitness doping policy and prevention have developed, as well as the ways in which fitness dopers view their practice in terms of individual choice. We argue that the USA and Sweden represent two extreme welfare state positions as depicted by Esping-Andersen's model, thus creating fertile ground for our analysis of fitness doping (cf. Rush, 2015). Taking the criticism expressed by scholars into account, we also move beyond Esping-Andersen's model in our analysis to capture some of the complexities of the international character of fitness doping.

One way of doing this is through the concept of *glocal*. While globalization often refers to a more general process, the term glocal explicitly addresses how national and local variations of supranational economic, cultural, and symbolic processes may occur (Urry, 2003). We will use the *glocal* concept to capture how global processes blend into and impact local patterns in gym and fitness culture, in general, and fitness doping, in particular. The fitness industry appropriates local traditions that are molded into new cultural and symbolic expressions, under the influence of both by global trends and the ideals of different welfare state regimes. Looking at fitness doping in a national comparative manner, we can thus see a combination of structural uniformity, where homogenization and power occur, and symbolic and localized diversity (Ram, 2004).

In relation to this discussion, in sections below, we will analyze how fitness doping is understood, transfigured, and treated within different national welfare regimes, as well as in relation to global sport and drug contexts. On a more abstract level, we will also touch on whether or not it is possible to discern and describe certain patterns and understandings of fitness doping as representations of transnational ideals and understandings within gym and fitness culture. However, the relationship between such hegemonic representations and ideals/understandings defined at national and local levels is understood to be complex, multi-layered, and sometimes contradictory (Elias & Beasley, 2009).

Individual Freedom and Doping in the USA

In the USA, doping substances are regulated under federal laws. The USA does not currently criminalize use at the federal level, but criminal penalties may be given for possession and trafficking. Substances are scheduled—placed into categories concerning their potential for medicinal use, abuse, and/or dependency—under the Controlled Substances Act (DEA, 2018). The Anabolic Steroid Control Act of 1990 (ASCA, 1990), as part of the Crime Control Act, expanded the Controlled Substances Act to include anabolic androgenic steroids. Steroids are Schedule III substances. According to the Drug Enforcement Agency, 'Schedule III drugs, substances, or chemicals are defined as drugs with a moderate to low potential for physical and psychological dependence' (DEA, 2018). The 1990 Act was in response to cheating scandals in sport, notably Ben Johnson's positive test at the 1988 Olympic Games (Denham, 1997). Years later, sparked by PIED use in professional baseball, the US Congress again held hearings and took up legislation to address doping (Denham, 2006). The Anabolic Steroid Control Act of 2004 (ASCA, 2004) further expanded the scheduled substances list to include hormone precursors (ethers, esters, salts), thereby increasing the number of banned substances from 23 to 59. The ASCA 2004 additionally installed new sanctions for falsely labeling products containing banned anabolic substances. Similarly, in 2014, the Designer Anabolic Steroid Control Act expanded the list to include substances 'structurally similar' to listed anabolic steroids, known as designer steroids (DASCA, 2014). As the focus of these laws tended to be on doping in professional, formally governed sport and trafficking issues, use among fitness dopers tended to slip through. Because many fitness dopers do not compete within organized sport contexts (including professional bodybuilding) and acquire substances for their own use, they may use a variety of substances without drawing the attention of any sport, police, or other enforcement agency, including WADA. This situation thus offers an environment in which users enjoy a kind of freedom to use.

As regards users' understandings and negotiations concerning fitness doping, one large mainstream US media outlet, *The New York Times*, has touched on the issue of steroids in two recent pieces on bodybuilders. One profiled former professional bodybuilder and now trainer Charles Glass. In the article, the author notes Glass's history with and view on steroids:

> He's not about to voice blanket opposition to performance-enhancing drugs. "I'd be a hypocrite," he said. He acknowledges the role steroids play with bodybuilders competing at the highest levels. But he does want clients using them to start making choices that factor in their health, including going to a doctor regularly and getting blood work done. (Bernstein, 2018)

This is reflective of harm-reduction approaches to substance use. In such an approach, the focus is on reducing health risk through information and support. The decision to use is left to the individual, while support and advice on safer use are made available without moral judgment (Stewart & Smith, 2008). A second profile focused on Phil Heath, who has won the Mr. Olympia contest six times. After describing Heath's workout and diet, the author described Heath's vagueness in response to a question about steroids and testing. The author notes that 'Fans of Mr. Olympia do not seem caught up in the issue, perhaps because the sport is entirely about aesthetics, not strength or performance' and then moves on (Branch, 2016). Though not the focus of either profile, steroid use is assumed and noted in both. The fact that fans are agnostic on the topic of doping points to a general understanding that steroids are part of the global bodybuilding scene, despite broader negative social attitudes toward doping in formally governed sport competitions.

The fact that use is so common and tolerated is highlighted in bodybuilding and fitness media and online forums. Some bodybuilding Web sites such as Bodybuilding.com offer information and debate about steroid use and its role in bodybuilding, but also make it clear that the site itself does not condone steroid use (Charlebois, 2017). Other fitness Web sites are more open to questions of use, such as Rxmuscle.com and T-nation.com, offering articles and information on how to most effectively use various steroid products, how to control side effects, and even tips on the best ways to procure substances. Each promotes individual choice and responsibility for use. One article by a professional bodybuilder, published under the Shadow Pro pseudonym, noted the open-secret nature of steroid use and how speculation misconstrues the issue:

Today things have changed, but I still hear a lot of lies and misconceptions about steroid use in professional, amateur, and "natural" bodybuilding. Most of this comes from online rumors and "gurus" throwing around nonsense. (Shadow Pro, 2015)

Shadow Pro goes on to lay out both the risks and the risk-reduction measures bodybuilders and others can take before outlining 16-week cycles for moderate to heavy use. The harm-reduction approach is evident in Shadow Pro's stated myth-busting and risk-reduction aims. Rather than ostracizing users or avoiding the issue altogether, members like Shadow Pro engage (potential) users as rational individuals who have chosen to use while empowering them to make the best decisions for their health. He understands, and presumably his readers do as well, that fitness doping is a reality in gym and fitness culture and that correct, harm-minimization information from within the fitness community will benefit fitness dopers.

New York-based Rxmuscle.com has a decidedly open view on steroid use and takes a harm-minimization approach in many articles. One feature on the multi-media site is 'Ask Dr. Blau,' in which Dr. Mordcai Blau answers questions from readers about gynecomastia, a possible side effect of steroid use. Similarly, under the forum for topics related to 'Chemical Enhancement, Science & Medicine' is a thread for 'Medical Q&A with Dr. Joel Nathan' (Nathan, n.d.), whose profile indicates he is a medical doctor with expertise in 'hormone replacement therapy for Age Management.' Nathan fields questions related to steroid use, side effects, and addiction in addition to supplements and nutrition. In response to one question about using a topical or injected testosterone, Nathan counsels:

Injections are the way to go. Topical testosterone gets converted to dihydrotestosterone (DHT) to a much greater degree than injections of testosterone. High DHT concentrations [sic] can increase prostate enlargement and baldness. (Nathan, 2014, August 20)

This provision of information and open attitude are consistent with the guiding ideas behind Rxmuscle.com, which it claims reflect 'the truth in bodybuilding.' It is also illustrative of the general acceptance of fitness doping observed in the USA. The fact that a for-profit company like Rxmuscle is offering harm-reducing advice directly to potential users is in line with neoliberal values. The responsibility for ensuring safe use is transfer from the state to the individual, creating a market for this information and any measures to counter unwanted effects (i.e., Esposito & Perez, 2014). Outlets like Rxmuscle provide this in exchange for page views and advertising, along with any services or products users may purchase as a result.

Bodies, as well as knowledge about how to chemically enhance them, are also commodified in the USA. When lean, muscled bodies are celebrated and idealized in consumer culture, people who achieve these results are normalized and celebrated as healthy (Dworkin & Wachs, 2009). Bodybuilders can craft non-normative bodies that may be viewed as freakish outside of bodybuilding spaces, but normal within them (Liokaftos, 2012). Producing those bodies, including the use of drugs, is in one respect the very core of bodybuilding culture. As the founder and central personality behind Rxmuscle David Palumbo notes, while steroid distribution is policed, fitness dopers are not penalized for appearing 'suspiciously' muscular. In an interview with Palumbo, conducted by the authors, he says the following regarding the situation in the USA, in comparison with Sweden:

> I think there's much more tolerance here, aside from anabolic steroids that they love to arrest people for, no one is like profiling people because they are big, and say let's arrest him 'cause he must be doing something wrong you know. In Sweden, you know they can arrest you if they think you are taking something or if you look too big. It's really bad. (David Palumbo)

Palumbo's observation links widespread beliefs about the built body and steroids to enforcement. As suggested above, steroid use (with regard to fitness doping) is fairly accepted in the USA and definitely more accepted than in Sweden. Built bodies are not criminalized or viewed as unhealthy, but instead seem to symbolize work to craft muscles and dedication to the pursuit by a variety of means. Enforcement of anti-doping laws in the USA focuses on distribution and trafficking rather than on personal use. This is in stark contrast to many views about the acceptability of recreational drug use and the provision of anti-drug education and prevention programs, as exemplified by the broader war on drugs and doping in formally governed sport (Henning & Dimeo, 2017).

Prevention strategies have largely targeted young people. Two doping-focused programs were the team-based Adolescents Training and Learning to Avoid Steroids (ATLAS) Program for male students and the Athletes Targeting Healthy Exercise & Nutrition Alternatives (ATHENA) Program for female students (Goldberg, Clarke, Green, Wolf, & Lapin, 1996). These programs combined classroom sessions with practical alternatives to steroid use. Though early evaluations were positive as regards reducing young people's interest in doping (Elliot et al., 2006), a meta-analysis revealed the programs had less impact on actual behavior (Ntoumanis, Ng, Barkoukis, & Backhouse, 2014). Apart from such school-based programs, most anti-doping education is handled through the United States Anti-Doping Agency (USADA). Such programs often miss the fitness demography/population, however. Anti-doping prevention tends to focus on formally governed and competitive sport contexts, teams, or the school environment rather than on the gym and fitness context, communities or spaces that adult fitness dopers are likely to engage with or frequent.

Fitness Doping as a Societal Problem in Sweden

Reports in the late 1980s showed that the use of doping in Swedish society had become an issue outside the sphere of formal competitive sport. Due to this, an investigation was initiated in 1989 in which the use of steroids and other chemical substances that increase the levels of testosterone in the human body was defined as both a societal problem and a severe public health issue. From a public health point of view, pressure was put on policymakers to do something in response. The result was a new law: the Swedish Doping Act (1991:969).

Unlike many other countries, Swedish law does not just prohibit the possession and trade of doping substances, but also the presence of these substances in the human body (cf. Pedersen, 2010; Christiansen, 2009). The Swedish Doping Act, adopted by the Swedish Parliament and brought into effect in 1992, made it possible to intensify anti-doping work by criminalizing use and possession of doping substances, and by implementing stricter criminal penalties. Following this development, public health organizations from the 1990s onwards contributed to the comprehensive anti-doping work being done in Sweden. As a result, in the public discourse, by policymakers, and in the research, doping has mainly been connected with crime, mixed abuse, and described in terms of deviance beyond a formally governed competitive sport context (see, e.g., Moberg & Hermansson, 2006). The framing of fitness doping as a social/societal problem has also meant that (ab)use has been incorporated into the Swedish educational system. To this end, there is an almost linear relationship between development of the Doping Act and institution of the Swedish anti-doping educational system. Beginning at the high school level, Swedish youth are educated on how to make sound and healthy choices in life, and on the health risks associated with drug use, including the use of PIEDs (Skolverket, 2011).

Due to this and other policy measures in Sweden, fitness doping has increasingly been marginalized in the public discourse and connected to physical decay, violence, and unhealthy lifestyles, among other negative attributes. This, of course, has also influenced users' understanding of the drugs and the ways in which their lifestyle choices are negotiated in relation to non-users. One Swedish user talks about his perception of fitness doping in relation to what he thinks is public opinion in Swedish society.

> I don't like being labeled as shabby. I mean you can have a bad reputation if you're a mean person, or have done something bad. But when you don't think that you have. I don't like it, being labeled as dirty. Today, they are likening a steroid, which makes your body's tissue heal a little faster, to other drugs. To me, these are two completely different worlds. (Markus)

Markus is expressing his irritation at how policymakers have come to connect use of PIEDs with drug addiction both through the Swedish school curriculum and through the public discourse (cf. Monaghan, 2001). According to him, this kind of representation makes his actual lifestyle choices invisible. He sees himself as a healthy person and works to distance himself from tobacco, alcohol, and narcotics. He exercises on a regular basis, but his experiences are shaped by the association with steroids caused by his muscular body. Another user, Louise, explained what happened to her one afternoon when leaving the gym after a training session:

> Well, I'm on my way to the car and these five civilian officers' approach me, 'give us your bag and phone, okay'. Yeah and they start asking questions, about steroids and things, and this was 3 weeks before competition. /.../ They had this really tough attitude when they picked me up, like I was the worst kind of thug. (Louise)

Louise depicts her lifestyle as being limited by Swedish state policy. Thus, as regards her bodybuilding practices, the political level is highly relevant at the individual level. Being a professional bodybuilder, Louise has also competed internationally, and she sees official policy and preventative measures in Sweden as far more rigorous and stricter than in many other countries. This view corresponds very well with Palumbo's thoughts presented earlier in the chapter. Adding to this, in both of the above narratives there is also an understanding that the (perceived to be) doped bodybuilding body is often stigmatized in Swedish society (Christiansen & Bojsen-Møller, 2012; Maycock & Howat, 2007). In relation to this, it is not surprising that 'new' ways to access fitness doping have emerged. In both the Swedish and transnational contexts, social media and Internet forums have become a means through which people can anonymously gain access to PIEDs.

In an online community called *Flashback*, for example, which describes itself as 'Sweden's largest forum for freedom of expression, opinion and independent thinking' (Flashback, n.d.), we find extensive discussions on prohibited activities including the use of PIEDs. In contrast to official national policy, here we are dealing with a somewhat virtual, subcultural, and glocalized arena where national prohibitions are contested (something we will return to in Chapter 6). However, there is a significant difference between discussing the use of PIEDs anonymously in an online forum and facing possible encounters with the police when going to the gym for a daily workout, as Louise experienced.

Preventative measures in Sweden can be understood as somewhat multifaceted. Great efforts have been made by the police and through mandatory prevention programs in the Swedish school curriculum. Additionally, the Swedish Sports Confederation coordinates and is the responsible organizing body for NADO in Sweden. It takes the lead in producing leaflets, newsletters, and videos as well as in organizing educational conferences. The official mission also requires collaborations with other organizations or agencies. One that has specialized in preventative work for fitness doping is the organization *Prevention of Doping in Sweden* (PRODIS), which is a co-operation between fitness centers and other stakeholders, aiming to support a doping-free gym and fitness environment. The most prominent intervention program of PRODIS is called '100% pure hard training.' From the program Web site:

> The main goal for the years to come is to spread this method to more training facilities in Sweden and to make more people cooperate in combating doping. We also want to develop the effectiveness, accessibility and feasibility of the method, and evaluate these aspects. One important part of the method is the interaction between various actors such as the police, prevention coordinators and training facilities [our translation]. (Prodis, 2018)

Currently, 28 municipalities in Sweden are connected to PRODIS. This community-based intervention program builds on a model originally developed for alcohol. Its intent is to establish local anti-doping plans and policies at different gyms, through a combination of educational components directed at managers and trainers at fitness facilities, and in co-operation with the Swedish Sports Confederation, the police, and media advocacy. A process through which training facilities can receive a diploma for promoting a drug-free environment is intended to link involved local actors together to create a national network and knowledge base that can be spread to other municipalities in the country. The operation of PRODIS builds on the idea of creating a set of values concerning doping, directed not only to doping users, but to all people operating within this context. As such, it is almost an archetypical example of what Esping-Andersen (1990) calls a social democratic welfare state model.

Comparing Policy, Practice, and Prevention

By comparing the cases of the USA and Sweden, we can see that anti-doping policies are developed within multiple contexts across various policy levels. The first context is the global level of formally governed and competitive sport. This is largely led by Olympic and international sport, but also includes organized professional sports outside the Olympic Movement. Sport in this context is heavily commercialized and spectacle driven. The highest profile doping scandals are usually at the most competitive levels. The second context is the hegemonic prohibitionist approach to drugs (e.g., the war on drugs). Within this context, all drugs outside the realm of serving medical needs are assumed to be dangerous and morally unacceptable, including PIEDs. Users of any illicit substance tend to be stigmatized. Global fitness culture is positioned within these two broader contexts, both shaping and being shaped by several levels of doping policy, practice, and prevention.

Anti-doping policies are determined and implemented across several levels. Policies are determined at the global level by two main bodies: WADA and the United Nations. Policies are refined, and possibly expanded, at the national level. Each country can pass anti-doping legislation to provide additional clarity for or assign responsibility to different stakeholders. Both the USA and Sweden have set up NADOs that work with national sport-governing bodies to implement global and national anti-doping policies. Implementation is thus predominantly directed at formally governed and competitive sport at local (national or sport group) levels, which largely leaves the fitness context out of the equation. The specific forms anti-doping has taken in the USA and Sweden align to some degree with Esping-Andersen's model. As a Nordic welfare state, Sweden tends to focus more on ensuring the common good. As such, Sweden's expanded anti-doping policies include non-formally governed sport contexts such as fitness centers through the connection between the NADO and the anti-doping organization PRODIS. Together with adoption of the Swedish Doping Act, this allows a legal mechanism to ensure that anti-doping policies are followed for the good of both the individual and society as a whole. In contrast, the USA is a liberal welfare state regime that prizes both individual responsibility and freedom, as well as less governmental control and regulation. Accordingly, the USA has taken an approach focused on criminal trafficking and fraud rather than on policing of individuals.

Fitness communities also exist across several different levels, as well as within both global and national contexts, subject to global and local laws and regulations. Online groups, forums, and media illustrate global fitness communities. Members of this broad community may share aesthetic ideals, training goals, methods, and substance use practices (licit and illicit). PIED use is broadly accepted as part of the culture, though views and use at the individual or local level are likely to vary. In practice, this means there may be little difference between Swedish and US fitness dopers' approaches to their training regimes and PIED use, because all are guided by globalized norms and ideals. However, Swedish users exist within a national context where other exercisers may view PIED use negatively, believing such practices break with global fitness norms. Swedish users may also face social sanctioning from those outside the fitness community, as individual PIED use is thought to damage the common good. This is exemplified by Swedish users' experience of being policed, often based on their non-normative musculature. Thus, in Sweden bodybuilding and civil/criminal contexts are conflated, resulting in civil policing of the fitness community as a whole. This local reality then informs and constrains individual choices regarding doping. In contrast, US fitness dopers are in a context where people inside and outside the local fitness community may disapprove of PIED use, but these dopers are unlikely to face any social consequences. Individual use—and health and safety—is viewed as the individual's responsibility. Because US fitness dopers are policed only if they enter formally governed competitions in sport contexts or in cases of criminal trafficking or possession, their use often has little external consequence, despite the widespread disapproval of sport doping.

Differences in prevention are also notable. As regards fitness doping, the Swedish prevention strategy is directly related to the national communal ethos. The primary goal of prevention is to encourage fitness athletes to police themselves, while turning the focus to non-drug-assisted methods of achieving improvement. This is possible due to the general social rejection of PIED use in Sweden and the high level of local enforcement of national strategies, where the Swedish Sport Confederation and PRODIS, in collaboration with local municipalities, work together to counteract fitness doping. The USA has little in the way of prevention among the adult fitness population. Instead, the more neoliberal US approach relies on criminal laws to deter trafficking or on anti-doping organizations to police athletes competing in formal competitions in sport contexts. US fitness enthusiasts and bodybuilders are thus unlikely to police one another as expected in the Swedish system, as PIED use is more widely tolerated, if not accepted. This results in little prevention among individual PIED users, who are left to make their own choices and take the consequences.

Conclusions

Fitness doping and anti-doping processes operate within multiple contexts and across various levels. This interplay between supranational structures and locally diverse implementation is not only complex, but can also seem contradictory, as each locality works to remain within the global system. The policies, practices, and prevention techniques found in national contexts can be partly explained using Esping-Andersen's model (1990, 2009): Sweden's Nordic welfare ethos is exemplified in policy and prevention methods that rely on social policing and public health, while the US approach sees use as a primarily individual choice and responsibility. However, we must consider the interplay between structured global systems and the more diverse local implementation. Fitness doping is generally tolerated, if not outright accepted or promoted, by the global fitness community, while doping in the global sports context is widely rejected. Global anti-doping policies and conventions are intended to deter use of PIEDs through prohibition and sanctioning. The countries considered here, Sweden and the USA, are governed by these global policies and exist within the global sport and drug context. Yet the implementation has been transfigured within the glocalized fitness context.

Anti-doping policies and intervention campaigns need to be understood within a framework of national and sometimes even local and community-based approaches to doping that affect how fitness doping is understood and approached by users as well as people operating in the field of anti-doping. The two national contexts/cases frame fitness doping and the notion of the doping user differently. At the same time, this chapter shows that there are some basic similarities both in the ways users negotiate the meaning of use and in transnational trajectories, such as within the context of online communication. What we suggest is that glocal fitness doping needs to be understood as a process through which global ideals, organizations, and more contribute to influencing local and national prevention policies and cultures, and vice versa. The contribution of this chapter thus lies in connecting the intersection of policies, practices, and prevention of fitness doping across local, national, and global levels. As shown by looking at two cases—the USA and Sweden—there is reason to believe that these levels are highly interconnected and dependent on each other, on the one hand, and that there is great national variation in how fitness doping is perceived and treated in terms of policy and anti-doping work, on the other. We suggest that there is a gap between the global and the local level that has largely been unaddressed by researchers and policymakers. To this end, and within this gap, the meaning and understanding of fitness doping has largely been negotiated within the context of the global fitness community, both online and off.

References

Andreasson, J. (2015). Reconceptualising the gender of fitness doping. Performing and negotiating masculinity through drug-use practices. *Social Sciences, 4,* 546–562.

Andreasson, J., & Johansson, T. (2014). *The global gym: Gender, health and pedagogies.* Basingstoke, UK: Palgrave Macmillan.

Andreasson, J., & Johansson, T. (2016). Online doping. The new self-help culture of ethnopharmacology. *Sport in Society: Cultures, Commerce, Media, Politics, 19*(7), 957–972.

ASCA. (1990). Public Law 101–647.

ASCA. (2004, March). Amendment to the Controlled Substances Act. 108th Congress; 2d Session; S. 2195.

Bambra, C. (2004). The worlds of welfare: Illusory and gender blind? *Social Policy and Society, 3*(3), 201–211.

Bambra, C. (2007). Going beyond the three worlds of welfare capitalism: Regime theory and public health research. *Journal of Epidemiological Community Health, 61*(12), 1098–1102.

Bernstein, J. (2018, January 3). Working out with Charles Glass, a trainer to the stars. *New York Times.* Retrieved from https://www.nytimes.com/2018/01/03/style/charles-glass-bodybuilder-workout.html.

Branch, J. (2016, October 28). No one is looking at this headline. *The New York Times.* Retrieved from https://www.nytimes.com/2016/10/29/sports/phil-heath-mr-olympia-bodybuilder.html.

Charlebois, D. (2017). *Taking steroids: What could it hurt?* Retrieved 10 October 2018 from https://www.bodybuilding.com/fun/teen-derek4.htm.

Christiansen, A. V. (2009). Doping in fitness and strength training environments. Politics, motives and masculinity. In V. Møller, M. McNamme, & P. Dimeo (Eds.), *Elite sport, doping and public health.* Odense: University Press of Southern Denmark.

Christiansen, A. V. (2018). *Motionsdoping. Styrketræning, identitet og kultur* [Recreational doping. Strength training, identity and culture]. Aarhus, Denmark: Aarhus Universitetsforlag.

Christiansen, A. V., & Bojsen-Møller, J. (2012). Will steroids kill me if I use them once? A qualitative analysis of inquiries submitted to the Danish anti-doping authorities. *Performance Enhancement & Health, 1,* 39–47.

DASCA. (2014). Public Law 113–260.

DEA. (2018). *Drug scheduling.* Retrieved from https://www.dea.gov/druginfo/ds.shtml.

Denham, B. E. (1997). Sports illustrated, the "war on drugs", and the Anabolic Steroid Control Act of 1990: A study in agenda building and political timing. *Journal of Sport and Social Issues, 21*(3), 260–273.

Denham, B. E. (2006). The Anabolic Steroid Control Act of 2004: A study in the political economy of drug policy. *Journal of Health & Social Policy, 22*(2), 51–78.

Dworkin, S. L., & Wachs, F. L. (2009). *Body panic: Gender, health, and the selling of fitness.* New York and London: New York University Press.

Elias, J., & Beasley, C. (2009). Hegemonic masculinity and globalization: 'Transnational business masculinities' and beyond. *Globalizations, 6*(2), 281–296.

Elliot, D. L., Moe, E. L., Goldberg, L., DeFrancesco, C. A., Durham, M. B., & Hix-Small, H. (2006). Definition and outcome of a curriculum to prevent disordered eating and body-shaping drug use. *Journal of School Health, 76*(2), 67–73.

Esping-Andersen, G. (1990). *The three worlds of welfare capitalism.* Cambridge: Polity Press.

Esping-Andersen, G. (2009). *The incomplete revolution.* Cambridge: Polity Press.

Esposito, L., & Perez, F. M. (2014). Neoliberalism and the commodification of mental health. *Humanity & Society, 38*(4), 414–442.

European Commission. (2014). *Study on doping prevention: A map of legal, regulatory and prevention practice provisions in EU 28.* Luxembourg: Publications Office of the European Union.

Flashback. (n.d.). *Flashback forum* [website]. Retrieved 9 October 2018 from https://www.flashback.org/.

Goldberg, L., Clarke, G. N., Green, C., Wolf, S. L., & Lapin, A. (1996). Effects of multidimensional anabolic steroid prevention intervention. *JAMA: The Journal of the American Medical Association, 276,* 1555–1562.

Hall, S., & Jefferson, T. (Eds.). (1976). *Resistance through rituals.* London, UK: Hutchinson.

Hanstad, D. V., & Houlihan, B. (2015). Strengthening global anti-doping policy through bilateral collaboration: The example of Norway and China. *International Journal of Sport Policy and Politics, 7*(4), 587–604. https://doi.org/10.1080/19406940.2015.1014394.

Hearn, J., & Pringle, K. (2009). *European perspectives on men and masculinities: National and transnational approaches.* London: Palgrave Macmillan.

Henning, A. D., & Dimeo, P. (2017). The new front in the war on doping: Amateur athletes. *International Journal of Drug Policy, 51,* 128–136. https://doi.org/10.1016/j.drugpo.2017.05.036.

Hoff, D. (2013). Dopning utanför idrotten – individualisering och muskulösa skönhetsideal. En studie av dopning i grundskola, gymnasium och på gym i Kalmar kommun. *Scandinavian Sport Studies Forum, 4,* 1–24.

Johnston, L. D., Miech, R. A., O'Malley, P. M., Bachman, J. G., Schulenberg, J. E., & Patrick, M. E. (2018). *Monitoring the future national survey results on drug use: 1975–2017: Overview, key findings on adolescent drug use.* Ann Arbor: Institute for Social Research, University of Michigan.

Liokaftos, D. (2012). *From 'classical' to 'freaky': An exploration of the development of dominant, organised male bodybuilding culture.* London: Goldsmith's College, PhD.

Maycock, B., & Howat, P. (2007). Social capital: Implications from an investigation of illegal anabolic steroid networks. *Health Education Research, 22,* 854–863.

McGrath, S., & Chananie-Hill, R. (2009). "Big Freaky-Looking Women": Normalizing gender transgression through bodybuilding. *Sociology of Sport Journal, 26,* 235–254.

Moberg, T., & Hermansson, G. (2006) *Mandom, mod och morske män. Anabola androgena steroider - medicinskt, rättsligt och socialt.* Göteborg: Mediahuset i Göteborg AB.

Monaghan, L. F. (2001). *Bodybuilding, drugs and risk: Health, risk and society.* New York: Routledge.

Monaghan, L. F. (2012). Accounting for illicit steroid use. Bodybuilders' justifications. In A. Locks & N. Richardson (Eds.), *Critical readings in bodybuilding* (pp. 73–90). New York, NY: Routledge.

Nathan, J. (2014, August 20). *Shots or gel for TRT? Thank you [Msg 6].* Retrieved 10 October 2018 from http://forums.rxmuscle.com/showthread. php?127992-Shots-or-Gel-for-TRT-Thank-You.

Nathan, J. (n.d.). *About me.* Retrieved 10 October 2018 from http://forums. rxmuscle.com/member.php?2279-Dr-Joel-Nathan.

Ntoumanis, N., Ng, J. Y., Barkoukis, V., & Backhouse, S. (2014). Personal and psychosocial predictors of doping use in physical activity settings: A meta-analysis. *Sports Medicine, 44*(11), 1603–1624.

Pedersen, I. K. (2010). Doping and the perfect body expert: Social and cultural indicators of performance-enhancing drug use in Danish gyms. *Sport in Society: Cultures, Commerce, Media, Politics., 13*(3), 503–516.

Pierson, C. (1998). *Beyond the welfare state.* London: Polity Press.

Pope, H. G., Kanayama, G., Athey, A., Ryan, E., Hudson, J. I., & Baggish, A. (2014). The lifetime prevalence of anabolic-androgenic steroid use and dependence in Americans: Current best estimates. *The American journal on Addictions, 23*(4), 371–377.

PRODIS. (2018). *100% ren hårdträning* [100% pure hard training]. Retrieved 10 October 2018 from: http://www.prodis.se/hem/metoden-100-ren-h% C3%A5rdtr%C3%A4ning.

Ram, U. (2004). Glocommodification: How the global consumes the local McDonald's in Israel. *Current Sociology, 52*(1), 11–31.

Rush, M. (2015). *Between two worlds of father politics: USA or Sweden?* Manchester: Manchester University Press.

Sassatelli, R. (2010). *Fitness culture: Gyms and the commercialisation of discipline and fun.* Basingstoke: Palgrave Macmillan.

Shadow Pro. (2015). *Steroids: What pro bodybuilders are really using.* Retrieved 16 June 2018 from https://www.t-nation.com/pharma/steroids-what-pro-bodybuilders-are-really-using.

Skolverket. (2011). *Läroplan, examensmål och gymnasiegemensamma ämnen för gymnasieskola.* Retrieved 27 August 2018 from: https://www.skolverket.se/undervisning/gymnasieskolan/laroplan-program-och-amnen-i-gymnasieskolan.

Smith, A. C. T., & Stewart, B. (2012). Body perceptions and health behaviors in an online bodybuilding community. *Qualitative Health Research, 22*(7), 971–985.

Statens Folkhälsoinstitut. (2011). *Dopning i Samhället* [Doping in society]. Östersund, Sweden: Statens Folkhälsoinstitut.

Stewart, B., & Smith, A. C. (2008). Drug use in sport: Implications for public policy. *Journal of Sport and Social Issues, 32*(3), 278–298.

The Swedish Doping Act. (1991:1969). *Dopningslagen.* Stockholm, Sweden: Svensk författningssamling SFS.

Urry, J. (2003). *Global complexity.* Cambridge: Polity Press.

Part II

Doping Trajectories

4

Images of (Ab)Users

Introduction

Naturally, being or becoming a fitness doper can have many meanings. It can involve a variety of motives, emotions, and ambitions, which can be expressed and understood in different ways. Statistical studies on doping prevalence and national differences in how use is understood can give us a glimpse into the ways in which men and women engage in doping practices—into how use is dealt with by structural conditions, preventative measures taken by the state, police work, educational campaigns, and more. To understand individual motives and trajectories, however, we need to do more than focus on numbers and discuss the health risks associated with use. We need to consider how the users themselves view the practices, their efforts to develop their bodies, and how they reach the goals they have set up for themselves. We also need to look at the emotional investments made in relation to use, and how they affect personal trajectories and social relations, among other things.

Starting from Part I, in which fitness doping has been contextualized broadly, in Part II we will let the reader become better acquainted with the fitness doping users who have contributed their stories. We present

© The Author(s) 2020
J. Andreasson and T. Johansson, *Fitness Doping*,
https://doi.org/10.1007/978-3-030-22105-8_4

four fitness dopers and describe their efforts to create something extraordinary through drug use practices. We also explore how these case studies represent different experiences of doping, training, family relations, and gender negotiations. When referring to our cases, we use the concepts of *narrative* and *narrative studies* (Smith & Sparkes, 2009). This is a way to mark the importance of every single narrative and every individuals' understanding of fitness doping, as well as a way to show how we have used the different stories we have studied. Although we have limited our use of prolonged case studies to this chapter, this perspective should be understood as representative of the book as a whole. As we see it, narratives constitute human realities and our modes of being; thus, they help guide action and are socioculturally shared resources that give substance and texture to people's lives (Sparkes & Smith, 2007). Put differently, narratives, or what also could be called storytelling, constitute an important aspect of people's efforts to make sense of their lives. What we aim to do in this chapter, and the chapters that follow, is to create a mosaic of different voices that can help us say something relevant about fitness doping experiences and understandings (Freeman, 2001).

In our first case, we meet Daniel, whose narrative accentuates the ambition to learn about the drugs, to become a bodybuilder and later a coach for others pursuing their bodily projects. This narrative also touches on relations with other family members. Next follows a case in which we become acquainted with Charlie and his experiences of investing heavily in a subcultural community of people like him and becoming part of a sort of secret society. Included here are also aspects of the physical decay associated with abuse and addiction, as well as a way out of a lifestyle that includes using performance- and image-enhancing drugs (PIEDs). In our third case, we will meet Christine, whose narrative exemplifies how the will to compete in fitness and later in female bodybuilding influences the choices made. Christine's narrative also exemplifies negotiations concerning fitness doping and gender. Finally, in our fourth case, we meet Julius, who is an occasional user. Julius has no plans of competing, but instead, this narrative gives us a glimpse of the rationale for recreational use that is intended to create a desirable body one can display/show off for others. The chapter ends with some concluding thoughts.

The Coach and Fitness Doper

Daniel is 35 years old and currently lives with his girlfriend in an apartment. The couple have no children, but recently, this issue has come up and they have started talking about raising a family. In their view, Daniel's lifestyle, including his daily workout routine, is somewhat difficult to combine with family life, so they have not yet decided on the issue. In daily life, Daniel works in an office within the media/IT sector. Almost every day after work, he goes to a nearby gym to work out. Training and muscle-building have been of great interest to him for many years. In his teens, however, he was more into soccer and wrestling, the latter initially getting him to go to a gym. He explains:

> I was young. You know, at that time you needed your parents' permission to train at a gym. But I continued to go there occasionally, to that gym. Then when I was about 19 or so, there was this bodybuilder who asked me if I wanted to go with him to a bodybuilding competition. I had no idea what to expect. I had no idea what bodybuilding was, and really wasn't into it in that sense. But I thought, 'why not.'

After accompanying the older bodybuilding friend to the competition, Daniel felt excited. He had not been into muscle-building practices for the kind of purposes he witnessed at the competition, and he was intrigued by this new experience. During this period, he lived at home with his parents, who supported him, preparing protein-rich diets and the like. Gradually, his interest in organized sports, i.e., soccer and wrestling, decreased, and by the time he was 20 years old, he was no longer involved in these sports. Instead, he focused on gym practices, and the idea of becoming a bodybuilder was developing. He was impatient, however, and before long he also wanted to know about doping and the possible effects of the drugs. In order to reach his goal, he decided to invest in a course of steroids.

> Actually, the first time, I bought the wrong stuff. I was young and I didn't know any better. The guy I bought the stuff from told me it was a certain kind of steroid, but it turned out to be something completely different. It was kind of a dangerous one, it was known to be dangerous. And I took it in really high dosages, but luckily, I didn't suffer from any side effects.

Nothing. I had no idea what I took, until afterwards. I mean its ignorance and as I said I was still young and learning.

During the years that followed, Daniel focused on learning more and more about how the body works and about the effects of doping. He also studied physiology and tried to find out, and understand, how the body is affected by different amino acids, peptides, steroids, diuretic, human growth hormones, insulin, and more. He read medical articles discussing muscular development and physiological possibilities and limitations. First and foremost, however, he tried to learn about steroids. In this process of learning and gaining experience, he also found new friends at the gym with whom he discussed courses, side effects, post-cycle therapy (PCT), and more. Adding to the contacts he had at the gym, he also became aware that he could get information from an unexpected person, namely his own mother, who was a medical doctor. The situation below is preceded by Daniel's mother finding steroids in his room.

> I remember it really well. She had placed it all on a silver plate in the kitchen, on the dining table. It's dead quiet in the room, when I come home, and usually it's like very cheerful and lively at home when we have dinner and so on. So, I come into the kitchen and see all my steroids there, on the table. I'm like 'okay'. My dad is dead quiet. He doesn't say anything. But my mother, she's like, 'what's this?' And I'm like, 'you know what that is.' 'Yes I do' she replies, 'but why haven't you talked to me about this.' I said 'nah I wanted to deal with that by myself.' Then she goes on, 'but I don't think you should take these'.......'I think you should take these other substances instead.' So, she actually recommended something that was less dangerous for me, healthier. Following that route, we developed a really good relationship and I kind of thought that I could ask my mom about anything. But I've also exploited her trust. She's a doctor and I've forged prescriptions for steroids so I could get them from pharmacies. I've exploited her trust and done some stupid shit too.

Daniel's mother obviously got upset when she found steroids in his room, but she also wanted to share her expertise in the area, not least to make sure her son did not take any unnecessary risks, and that he understood the possible consequences of being involved in this kind of drug use practice.

The confrontation seems to have changed their relationship, in what Daniel describes as 'kind of a twisted way.' They began talking about PIED use, both in theory and in practice, and to this end, his mother has both discouraged and advised him. Following this situation, Daniel wanted to 'try everything' for a couple of years, and he used his body as a canvas for experimentation. He was not totally honest with his mother about the magnitude of his use, but still, he tried to keep her informed, especially so he could get 'inside information' on choice of steroids, risks, and more. He explains that he has experienced few serious side effects, but mentions nerve twitches, acne, and a completely torn breast muscle. He has also been arrested and convicted for selling steroids, which can be seen as an unwanted side effect of his involvement in doping.

Owing to his more than fifteen years of involvement in the business, Daniel has also become quite notorious in the social circles of bodybuilding and body fitness. Today, he is a well-known and respected person in the steroid business world in Sweden. Although he initially had plans to compete as a bodybuilder, he now coaches others, both bodybuilders and fitness competitors. Currently, he is trying to decide whether or not he should quit his work at the office and go for this new career. He says:

> So, I've started thinking about this, as a possible future career. And I'm like this grey zone coach. I make all kinds of schedules you know, as I have become quite knowledgeable in medicine as well. And this is something I struggle with every day. Yeah if someone comes up and asks me if I could make them a program. He pays me for that, and then comes the question about doping, which makes me a bit hesitant. I mean it's illegal, right. It feels contradictory. Should I help them and share my knowledge? What if they misuse this knowledge and do something stupid? And I meet these young guys who lack experience and have never used before, and I certainly wouldn't recommend that they start.

Daniel's approach to doping has changed over time. Initially, he wanted to be competitive in wrestling, and later this developed into a desire to become a bodybuilder. He invested heavily in drug use practices to reach the latter goal. Today, however, he mostly looks at himself as a coach and muscle-building guide. He still talks about competing now and then, but it seems he is not really dedicated to following this career path at present.

Instead, he enjoys the attention and respect he receives from others as a coach.

One thing that worries him, however, is the increasing trafficking of steroids and other kinds of drugs over the Internet. He suggests that discussing and dealing with doping over the Internet creates a dangerous distance between the person who knows the products and has the knowledge and the person who is buying them with the intent to use. To deal with this development, he explains that he always makes a great effort to get to know his trainees, trying to take some degree of responsibility for their health and well-being. Currently, his own goals concerning training are to stay fit and have a 'representable' body that corresponds with his coaching skills; achieving these goals includes occasional use of steroids and human growth hormones.

Charlie and the Secret Society

Another fitness doper we met during the research process is Charlie. He is currently 49 years old and became involved in bodybuilding as a teenager. In 1987, he qualified to compete in bodybuilding, so it is fair to say that he, like Daniel, invested highly in muscle-building practices during adolescence. In his twenties, he moved from a small city in southern Sweden, where he lived with his parents and two sisters, to the capital of Sweden, Stockholm. Soon he was spending more or less all his free time at the gym. He describes his training schedules and lifestyle in vivid detail and also talks about his fascination with muscles, symmetry, and bodybuilding. Charlie describes himself as something of a restless adventurer, who wants to travel and experience things. Before long, his adventure-seeking behavior also came to involve PIED use. When talking about his first experiences of the drugs, he is excited and describes discovering a 'new world.'

> It was really exciting as well, really. So, I think, partly, you'll get a pretty big placebo effect too. You know, 'wow, now I'm taking these pills, and I'm going to become really huge,' which makes you work out even harder. I gained weight, became stronger and also recovered faster. It was a bit like

that. I had my own box with the stuff, it was my treasure. It was the same when you visited someone, and he had his own box, and you looked in the box. It was like small treasure boxes. Your secret treasure!

Charlie explains how he gradually became part of gym culture and the bodybuilding subculture. He spent enormous amounts of time at the gym, among other bodybuilders. He also describes this as a learning process; he learned more and more about training schedules, methods, and, of course, steroids. This is thus a process of 'becoming,' a process through which a certain lifestyle develops. It is also a process of identity formation, finding oneself, establishing a self, creating a body, and so on. Charlie continues:

> At this time, there were lots of things going on. I'm especially thinking about what you asked about before, concerning my motivation to work out, but it becomes your identity, really, a lifestyle. I followed a tight time schedule, and weighed the food and yes, I worked a couple of years, selling food supplements and so on. I travelled to different gyms and so on. Competitions were also something, it was also big, yes. I met that guy from Gothenburg, and it was really such a community feeling, a world of its own.

For a couple of years, Charlie was completely involved in bodybuilding. He had some success, and he also felt a sense of belonging to a community, a brotherhood. He describes this as becoming part of a very special, secluded world.

> But as you put it, it's this classic feeling, you get stuck, and you also develop a sense of belonging to something, to the gym. Also, at the gym there was this tight, small group, doing drugs. Yes, it's interesting, you understand each other much better; someone might be annoyed that day, and then you knew that it could be really shaky when you're on a course of steroids or something. You knew, yes, shit he's into it a lot now, then we just knew, don't disturb him. It was a signal that you learned to understand, it was all part of the game. It's kind of funny.

Charlie describes how he was drawn into a subcultural space, where specific rules and social regulations applied. Everything soon revolves around courses, steroids, and training schedules. In this particular space, a certain language, style, and habits develop, and members of the group make great efforts to maintain solidarity through non-verbal, mutual understanding.

After a couple of intensive years, where Charlie put all his efforts and aspirations into bodybuilding, he became painfully aware of the negative aspects of his lifestyle. His relationship with his girlfriend, Sarah, broke down. Suddenly, he was alone, and he started feeling bad about his self-consuming lifestyle. In this process, he also turned his interest to other drugs and, as he describes it, he developed an addiction. To him, the step from taking steroids to including other drugs was not very great. Trying to deal with his life situation, he used amphetamines, cocaine, and also consumed quite a bit of alcohol. Soon, however, he realized that something needed to be done and that he had to veer off this established path/trajectory. He moved away from Stockholm and stopped going to the gym for a while, deciding not to touch drugs of any kind. Reflecting on this, he says:

> I met some of my old friends, afterwards. My whole world fell apart. I didn't visit the gym again for a while, because I felt I didn't want to get into it all again. We sat down and had a meal, I told him that I was really in trouble two years ago, and he told me that he understood that something had happened. But I got back on track again. He said it's too bad this. Then he told me he couldn't stop taking the steroids. He didn't want to lose weight, like the withdrawal. One can get stuck that way too.

Charlie's exit process from steroids and bodybuilding, as well as other drugs, was successful, although it came at a high price. He lost the woman he still describes as the love of his life. And he repeatedly talks about this previous relationship and what could have been. Sarah now has a family with kids and a new man, and he is by himself. He also struggles with anxiety and worries about falling back into addiction. Leaving the comradeship and the bodybuilding scene was also painful. Today, Charlie has returned to the gym, and he works out regularly two or three times a week. He is not involved in competitions, and he is drug-free.

Christine and the Gender Balance

Christine is 28 years old. She comes from a family that she describes as having a more laid-back and sedentary way of life, and thus, she has no sporting background. In her late teens, however, she started occasionally visiting a nearby gym in the small village in which she lived and had grown up. At that time, there were not that many women in the gym environment, except for a few group training activities. Christine initially focused on aerobics, but gradually, she became interested in body fitness and weight-training. She describes how she felt at home in the gym. Having, or rather making, a muscular body was seen as something 'natural' there, whereas muscles and femininity, according to her, were regarded as opposite things in everyday life outside the gym. She started competing in body fitness in 2012, and some years later she had advanced to body-building. Since then, Christine has switched between body fitness and bodybuilding, depending on how she has related to her body. She also describes the transition from being in competitive mode and returning to everyday life as quite problematic.

> I have one body when competing, and another when it's time for off-season training. Most of the competitors start eating after their competitions. Therefore, after a few weeks, you look like someone else, and then you return to your normal state, you know, so you get a little more meat on your bones, fatter, and so on. Sure, it's like that. You have two different bodies. I usually say that you have two different wardrobes, you know, one for the off-season and one for getting in shape for the competitions again.

Christine talks a lot about how she perceives her body. On the one hand, working out and lifting the weights are understood as liberating, a way to construct a competent and admirable body. She struggles hard to gain muscle mass and change her body in accordance with the demands of the judges and the body fitness culture. On the other hand, she also relates to other ideals and the desire to fit into what she describes as a 'normal life.' Although she has a certain distance to gym and fitness culture and its masculinized body ideals, she also finds that she is part of this world. Negotiating gender and the meaning of muscular bodies is understood as quite complex and dependent on the particularities of the socio-spatial environment. Christine explains:

> I mean most people have told me that when I competed in bodybuilding, after fitness, and to this day, that I still have a feminine face. Most women doing bodybuilding don't have that. When they gain lots of muscle mass they usually do it because they've used certain drugs you know, making them muscular and look manly. But to me, building muscles is fairly easy, and therefore I can also be fairly modest concerning the drugs. Also, you can accomplish things through training hard alone. Therefore, I can keep this female thing, femininity. /.../ I can imagine doing other types of operations also, beauty surgery. I cannot imagine what I will think about this in say ten years' time. If I would think, 'I should not have made my breast that huge' or 'I should not have used Botox,' for example. Therefore, clearly it's not that good for your self-image, entering into this fake world. Still, it's the surface you are molding and shaping.

Although she invests a great deal in muscle-building practices and fitness doping, Christine does not want to look like a bodybuilder, or maybe more correctly, she has occasionally wanted to be perceived as a bodybuilder, but she is also aware of the cultural association between muscles and masculinity. Lately, she has chosen to compete in body fitness. Just as in the case of Charlie's secret society, she talks about two different worlds: one muscle-building community and one ordinary or mainstream world, which is mainly, but not exclusively, understood as situated outside the fitness context/culture. She suggests that many female bodybuilders have chosen the gym setting, as their place of belonging. Crafting an 'edgier' and rougher muscular appearance, however, is not one of her goals. Instead, she pursues a perspective on the body that makes 'dual citizenship' possible. Concerning female bodybuilders:

> I think it's a bit of an exaggeration. They've ended up in this world (*Read: Bodybuilding*), and they've left the other world. They're only in this world now and they don't care what others think. That's also wrong. I want to have the kind of look that I can be like a chameleon; you can fit in in the normal world, but you can also fit in in this world.

Christine is not particularly happy about talking about doping and drugs. When bringing the subject up, she tries to explain it as a more or less 'natural' part of gym and fitness culture, not least as concerns the more competitive aspects of muscle-building. She also compares doping with alcohol and brings up the notion of an individual choice. In line with neoliberal values, and the cult of the individual, norms concerning doping are challenged and the possible consequences of use are simultaneously placed on the individual. She tries to explain how things can get out of hand, but not if you are prepared to take responsibility for your actions.

> As I always say, it's your own body, and some people choose to use alcohol and destroy their homes and stuff. Certainly, you harm the public, because we, the taxpayers, have to pay for it. However, I believe that it's still my body, and I'll do it if I want to. As long as I don't kill someone. In the media, everyone using doping substances is described as crazy. This is simply not true, but some people who consume alcohol become addicts, of course. Therefore, everything has two sides. I don't believe in creating a moral panic around this. In that case, things are merely escalating.

This discussion on moral panic and the media understanding of doping users as 'crazy' should probably be understood within a Swedish context, where strong preventative measures have been aimed at fitness dopers. As argued in Chapter 3, internationally there are 'good' examples of more forgiving attitudes, even cultural acceptance, in other countries, such as the USA. Nevertheless, Christine is deeply involved in fitness doping, but at the same time, she is trying to uphold what she thinks is a more 'normal' lifestyle. She does not want to become a bodybuilder fully, not in the sense that she understands this position anyway. She does not want to invest in drug use practices and bodybuilding to such an extent that she 'risks' losing what she understands as her femininity or a body that connotes femininity. She also describes how certain women become masculine and 'lose' their (feminine) appearances. She is clearly balancing between being a successful competitor in body fitness, molding her body and using an adequate amount of drugs, and living an 'ordinary' life with work, family, and friends outside the cultural sphere of the gym and fitness.

Side Effects and Youth Prevention

Julius is 25 years old and has always been into sport, living an active lifestyle. When he was about 18 years old, he visited a gym for the first time and did not particularly care for the training done there. Nevertheless, he and some friends started working out a couple of days a week, mainly using different machines, but they also did circuit training and spinning. After two years of going to the gym, however, upon turning 20, he could not see any results or not good enough results anyway. Among his peers, there had been talk about and use of different supplements for quite some time, and Julius always had a protein shake with him when he went for a workout. But he felt that something more was needed and, therefore, decided to initiate a course of PIEDs. He explains:

> And to me it was not about competing in bodybuilding or something like that, not at all. It was more, I think, about boosting my self-esteem, you know, to get a nice body for the upcoming beach season. I wanted to be better looking, so to speak. And there were also these guys who took it as a kind of a sex drug, because they'd heard that you could get bloody horny.

Julius had no ambition to become a competitive bodybuilder. Instead, he did lots of circuit training and spent hours on the treadmill. Moreover, he 'only' used PIEDs occasionally, most often in the springtime to ensure a more attractive, fitter body for the beach. Good looks were important to him, and seemingly, there were also other motives for drug use among Julius' friends. However, Julius explains that he felt somewhat hesitant about his drug use practices. He found it difficult to square his thoughts about living a healthy and ordinary life with the courses of illicit drugs he had at home.

> You train to be healthy and then you do this. You take all these substances that kind of work in the opposite direction, in a way. But you don't realize that, there and then. These side effects. You know, anything can happen, but I kind of thought 'Nah, that won't happen to me.' Still, it was always there, that feeling. And only to give an example, the first thing I did when I got off the steroids was to book an appointment to check my sperm count, to see that everything was alright down there. Why did I do that? Of course

because I had been worried about not being able to become a father one day. Still I kind of told myself, 'Nah, it won't happen to me.' You kind of suppress it.

Although he often felt worried about his doping practices, Julius continued to take occasional courses of PIED. When he turned 23, however, he told his friends that he wanted to stop using. They were mostly supportive of his decision, because he had explained that he no longer felt at ease with it. And they had their own training to focus on. Julius had also experienced some side effects:

> I kind of wanted out of the whole situation, and then I got these bitch tits. You know gynecomastia, and had to have surgery for that later. That was another thing your mates told you, 'It's not gonna be a problem, there are things for that too.' 'You only need to take this and that.' But it didn't work for me so I had to operate. And all this stuff you take, I had no idea. I only got it and kind of thought 'excellent and perfect.' Now, looking back at it everything seems strange. I kept one of the blister packs with pills and called the anti-doping hot line to ask about it. It turned out to be this breast cancer medicine that you give to women with breast cancer, and I kind of took that. Supposedly it works for some. But it did not work for me.

Being a fairly modest user, Julius has experienced some troubles and side effects with his fitness doping practices. Some of his friends have been more heavily involved, but according to him, they have experienced far less side effects. To this end, Julius views his 3-year-long period as a fitness doper as having been very unfortunate. After deciding to stop doping, he also tried to understand what had happened to him, his body, and why he had engaged in the practice in the first place. Once he visited a seminar on doping, organized by the municipality he lived in. This seminar was part of an anti-doping campaign, and there was a great deal of information on youth at risk and how doping had become a health problem for young people. Julius could identify with much of what was said. He talked with police officers in attendance and two nurses from the anti-doping hotline. In a way, this occasion seems to have been the starting point for a career choice. Julius felt he had some important experiences he wanted to share, in some way. So he applied to a university and was recently accepted by the department of education, focusing on physical education. Teacher training allows him to interact with pupils, not so much younger than he was when he got involved with doping. He explains what these interactions have brought:

> So, I spend a lot of time at the university, but there are also these parts of my education when you go out to a school, with this supervisor, and kind of follow him in his daily work, meeting the pupils. You know acting like a teacher or trying to be one. I'm at this school, and we have this information on doping. My supervisor tells the pupils about doping and unhealthy lifestyles, and there is this silence in the room. The pupils listen, and I realize that they really have no idea. But still there are many young people who take steroids you know. And particularly those who are about to become physical education teachers will meet these youngsters, mostly boys, because I guess there are not that many girls who do this. But I think one big problem today is the body ideals.

Today, Julius has stopped using steroids. He talks about his previous experiences in terms of both social inclusion/camaraderie and solidarity and risks and unwanted side effects. He still trains regularly, but is now more interested in his educational career and the process of becoming a physical education teacher. As a teacher, he hopes to make some contribution to young people's lives. His previous experiences have thus been transformed, for example, the stigma carved into his body in the form of scaring tissue after the gynecomastia surgery has turned into sort of a capital that can be used for doping prevention.

Variations in Fitness Doping

The case studies presented and discussed in this chapter were selected to represent some of the variety found in the narratives this book is based on. Our ambition was to bring the reader into the book's focus on fitness dopers' narratives on doping, the body, gender, social relations, and sense of subcultural belonging. We also wanted to present an extended illustration of the complexity of the narratives and fitness doping trajectories that we have gathered through interviews and observations. As shown, there are many different ways to approach and possibly leave a lifestyle that includes the use of PIEDs. This is partly a consequence of our limited material, but it also reflects actual structural differences in how doping is understood in relation to normative gender configurations, national legislation, and subcultural affiliations. Departing from such structural conditions, scholars have often aimed at constructing typologies that can identify illicit drug users and their motives. Although this research is highly valuable, here we have tried to instead present our narratives on a more subjective level, aiming to capture some of the complexities and continuous movements that these four narratives represent. At the same time, some core similarities also emerge, and we will return to them in the chapters that follow.

In the first part of the book, we painted a broad picture of the historical development of gym and fitness culture, in general, and fitness doping, in particular. These developments and cultural transformations are also nonlinear to a certain extent and characterized by constant backlashes. Neither normative gender patterns in society nor the development of legislative measures is enough to change how women and men understand doping and how their doping practices are incorporated into their everyday lives, which consist of training and drug using practices, but also family life, work, social relations, and more. Instead, a great variety of circumstances influence an individual's doping trajectory: a new job, new friends, inclusion in or exclusion from a particular sociocultural context or a specific event in a person's life, changing gender ideals, health issues, and so on. To this end, the relationship between social structures and the individual and his/her doped body is dialectical and complex, and it needs to be understood in relation to the particularities of the temporospatial context.

In presenting these four cases, we have tried to incorporate some of this dialectic into our narrative approach, not least to show how understandings of the self and the body change over time and take place on a social arena, formed in relation to social encounters, cultural contexts, and feelings of belonging. A body in transition, owing to drug use practices, can in a sense be understood almost linguistically. Bodies talk. They express things, such as cultural affiliations, gender, identities, and lifestyle choices; they are performative, they learn, and they have directions and intents, although this is not always explicitly experienced or thought of by the 'bearer.' In the chapters that follow, we will further develop our line of reasoning concerning these issues, focusing on our understanding of fitness doping trajectories, gender and health. Although staying true to our narrative approach to the data, we will not present additional extended case studies. Instead, we will let the many voices and experiences of the fitness dopers we have interviewed be heard.

References

Freeman, M. (2001). Worded images, imaged words: Helen Keller and the poetics of self-representation. *Interfaces, 18,* 135–146.

Smith, B., & Sparkes, A. C. (2009). Narrative inquiry in sport and exercise psychology: What can it mean, and why might we do it? *Psychology of Sport and Exercise, 10*(1), 1–11.

Sparkes, A. C., & Smith, B. (2007). Narrative constructionist inquiry. In J. A. Holstein & J. F. Gubrium (Eds.), *Handbook of constructionist research* (pp. 295–314). New York: The Guilford Press.

5

(Un)Becoming a Doping User

Introduction[1]

Although the scholarly debate has mainly focused on doping in sport (Dimeo, 2007; Mottram, 2005; Waddington, 2000; Waddington & Smith, 2009), research on doping among the general public, most often understood as taking place in the context of gym and fitness culture, has expanded significantly in recent decades (Brennan, Wells, & Van Hout, 2017; Liokaftos, 2017; Mogensen, 2011; Monaghan, 2001). From being considered almost an exclusively male preoccupation with certain typical features, such as positive attitudes toward doping (DuRant, Escobedo, & Heath, 1995; Klein, 1993; Locks & Richardson, 2012; Monaghan, 2001), the notion and demography of gym and fitness culture have shifted, widening into a popular enterprise (Sassatelli, 2010). Currently between 10 and 15% of the population in most Western countries exercises regularly at a fitness facility, and in segments of the young adult population,

---

[1] Some passages in this chapter have previously been published in Andreasson and Johansson (2014). They have been modified to fit into the present text/chapter.

the proportion is considerably higher (Andreasson & Johansson, 2014; IHRSA, 2016).

The widespread availability of doping and its growing prevalence among mainstream fitness groups have contributed greatly to the recognition of an emergent public health issue, which has been addressed internationally (Christiansen, 2009; Christiansen, Schmidt Vinther, & Liokaftos, 2016; McNamee et al., 2014; Van Hout & Hearne, 2016). As suggested by Brennan et al. (2017), the scholarly debate has paid surprisingly little attention to understanding fitness doping trajectories. Consequently, the pathways to and from doping in the gym and fitness context have not been sufficiently documented, at least as regards doping trajectories outside the sphere of competitive bodybuilding (Brennan et al., 2017). Aligning with this, in this chapter we describe and analyze the processes involved in becoming and unbecoming a fitness doping user.

We argue that this knowledge is of great importance, as it deals with the trajectories of individual subjects and how their perceptions of health, gender, the self and the body change over time. Arguably, this knowledge also represents an important starting point for the development of doping-prevention strategies (a discussion initiated in Chapter 3). We explore in what ways the participants' sporting background and introduction to the gym and doping can be described and understood, and in what ways the narratives can be analyzed in terms of exit processes. Throughout the chapter, we gradually close in on the question of how the processes of becoming and unbecoming a fitness doping user can be understood analytically, a discussion that will also be touched on in the concluding chapter.

The structure of the chapter is as follows: Initially, the general background of the chapter is explained in relation to how researchers have, in different ways, addressed the question of doping trajectories as well as processes of unbecoming a fitness doper. This is followed by a short discussion of conceptual choices and how we analytically understand processes of (un)becoming in the chapter, as well as generally in this part of the book. Next follow several sections in which narratives from fitness doping users are presented, and we discuss their fitness doping trajectories.

Finally, in the concluding section, we bring the discussion together in a more summative manner.

Engaging and Disengaging—A Short Background

Research on doping 'triggers' and doping trajectories is scarce (Brennan et al., 2017). Initially, in the 1990s and early 2000s, the existing debate on and analysis of the paths to becoming a fitness doper tended to lean heavily on individual and psychosocial perspectives (Lucidi et al., 2008). Hence, during this period, epidemiological and structural functionalist perspectives, typically employing quantitative measures, were (and to some extent still are) predominant. Using regression analysis, researchers identified male gender, the use of other drugs (including alcohol), and strength training as significant predictors of people's engagement in, and to some extent disengagement from, fitness doping (DuRant et al., 1995; Lucidi et al., 2008; Zelli, Lucidi, & Mallia, 2010). In a similar vein, Sagoe, Andreassen, and Pallesen (2014) conducted a systematic review and synthesis of qualitative literature on the trajectory and etiology of steroid use. Their results indicated that achieving enhanced sports performance, an enhanced appearance and increased muscle bulk/strength are key motives behind the initiation of steroid use, which usually takes place before the age of 30. Regarding people's ways of disengaging from the use of prohibited substances, scholarship in the field has focused mainly on attitudes toward doping and on how knowledge about such attitudes can be used to develop preventative measures. Nilsson, Spak, Marklund, Baigi, and Allebeck (2005) conducted a cross-sectional survey ($n = 4049$) of secondary schools in Sweden. Not surprisingly, having concluded that non-users' and users' attitudes toward doping differ in several respects (regarding, e.g., perception of masculinity, muscularity, and drugs), they suggested that these differences should be taken as a point of departure when designing complex intervention programs (see also, European Commission, 2014).

On the one hand, the above-described research has contributed greatly to framing our understanding and knowledge of doping. On the other hand, the tools provided by this research often tend to be somewhat blunt—being capable of identifying risk factors, but unable to fully capture the processes and complexities of individual narratives and trajectories. Obviously, far from all men engage in illicit drug use, although male gender has been recognized as a doping drive/trigger. Voices have also been raised arguing for the need to broaden our approach to the issue. Thualagant (2012) stressed the need to reconceptualize and revitalize our approach to fitness doping, including more sociologically informed perspectives on aspects such as body-enhancing techniques, anti-doping strategies, and fitness doping in relation to gender and identity (see also, Andreasson, 2015). Somewhat continuing this line of thought, Christiansen et al. (2016) concluded that media portrayals, as well as some research, tend to offer skewed, simplistic, and sensationalist pictures of steroid users (Bell, Buono, & Rawady, 2009). They suggested that if we are to establish effective educational anti-doping campaigns and prevention programs, we must have a nuanced understanding of the target population (see also, Kimegård & McVeigh, 2014). Aiming to widen the debate, they offered a heuristic tool in the form of a theoretically informed typology consisting of four general types of users: the Expert type, the Well-being type, the YOLO type, and the Athlete type. As regards *the Expert type,* involvement in fitness doping is understood as part of what could be termed an applied science project. In many cases, this is based on a fascination with the effects of pharmacological substances on human physiology as well as the knowledge one can acquire and control one can have over one's own body (p. 3). *The Well-being type* is less results-oriented, takes few risks, and is more interested in using doping to look and feel good. Then, we have *the YOLO type* ('you only live once'), who embraces risky behavior in the pursuit of new experiences and excitement. This type feels one should enjoy life fully even if that entails going over one's limits (p. 5). Finally, there is *the Athlete type,* whose primary reason for engaging in drug using practices is to prepare for and perform at competitions, often exemplified by competitor bodybuilders, but also including fitness competitors, powerlifters, strongmen, and others. Although there is considerable variation both across and within the types, they nevertheless can be used as heuristic tools to capture some of the variations in users' approaches to fitness doping. This somewhat diversified view of fitness dopers has also been echoed in a few qualitative studies.

One of the most influential papers in this area was written by the British sociologist Lee Monaghan (2001), who conducted a long-term ethnographic study on bodybuilders' drug using practices and risk nego-tiations. The results of that study further elucidate the variation in fitness doping experiences, reasons for commencing doping, and nego-tiations concerning the meanings attached to drug use practices (see also Kimegård, 2015; Sagoe et al., 2014). Whereas Monaghan's study stressed mainly, but not exclusively, the importance of carnal, psycho-logical and social factors/dimensions in individuals' initiation of doping, others have approached the field from a cultural and sociological per-spective. Liokaftos (2018) studied the development of natural—that is, drug-free—bodybuilding as a distinct body culture within bodybuild-ing. Situated within a broader historical development, the emergence of natural bodybuilding is sketched as a trajectory within the broader phe-nomenon of performance- and image-enhancing drugs (PIEDs). In doing so, Liokaftos contributed to the dissolution of overly simplified public conceptions of fitness doping, in general, and of bodybuilding—as a sub-cultural enterprise associated with doping—in particular.

Trajectories, Identities, and Doping

This chapter, and the part of the book consisting of Chapters 4–6, takes a cultural sociological approach to the question of fitness doping trajectories. What we are interested in is the intersubjective ways in which individuals learn about, approach, and subsequently distance themselves from fitness doping, through processes of socialization in a given cultural context. This discussion was initiated in the previous chapter, where we became acquainted with a few fitness dopers and their experiences, and it will be more systematically developed in this chapter and the next. As touched on, engaging in, as well as disengaging from, fitness doping can be understood in different ways, and as something that 'happens' over time, in relation to social encounters, through bodily practices and in relation to different cultural contexts. This means that the concept of *trajectory*, as we use it, is understood as being tightly interwoven with the concepts of *identity* and *learning processes*. Inspired by the words of Becker, we argue that drug use:

/.../ is the result of a sequence of social experiences during which the person acquires a conception of the meaning of the behavior, and perceptions and judgments of objects and situations, all of which make the activity possible and desirable. Thus, the motivation or disposition to engage in the activity is built up in the course of learning to engage in it and does not antedate this learning process. (Becker, 1953, p. 235)

Aiming to describe and analyze processes of engaging in and disengaging from a particular practice, the challenge lies in the possibility to both theoretically and empirically capture different sets of changes that occur in pre- and post-use individuals' ways of conceptualizing and experiencing doping use. Another way of looking at this relates to Ebaugh (1988) and her thinking on exit processes (which we understand here as possibly including the process of commencement of and exiting from doping practice). Ebaugh uses the idea of stages, the first stage of the role exit—the *doubting stage*—occurring when the individual starts to question a certain role commitment, which may occur for different reasons. The doubting stage is characterized by a reinterpretation of meanings and a critical attitude toward the role. The next stage is defined by a *search for alternatives.* At this point, an exploration of alternative ways of living and thinking is initiated. As part of the process of weighing alternatives, individuals at this point also begin to rehearse, learn about, and try out new positions. Stage three is *the turning point.* There are five major types of turning points, according to Ebaugh: specific events, time-related factors, excuses, either/or alternatives, and what she calls 'the straw that broke the camel's back' (p. 125). *Specific events* can be deaths in the family or other emotionally charged moments in life. Many role exits can be related to *time*, that is, the individual's age, and so on. The last stage, *creating an ex-role*, is characterized by the struggle to create a new life.

This type of stage-based model has been heavily criticized. Basically, the argument is that it is impossible to use these kinds of preconceived stages to map out an individual's life (Burman, 2008). Altier, Thoroughgood, and Horgan (2014) highlighted the importance of taking a flexible approach to exit processes. In order to complement and revitalize theories of disengagement, we suggest there is a need to connect to theories of subcultures. To study subcultures, we need to contextualize and address both the complex and contradictory structure and content of these cultures, as well as the hierarchical relations involved in organizing subcultures. We propose that entry into and exit from a *subcultural space*—that is, a social, cultural, and material context defined by certain values, behaviors, attitudes, and taste cultures—also marks the transition into a period of life in which the young aspirants become involved in several defining actions and ways of thinking about life (see also Chapter 1) (Johansson, 2017).

Adding to this, and inspired by Halberstam's (2005) analyses of queer transitional processes, we suggest that it is important to try to define and reflect on what it means to enter into and exit from a subcultural practice. Applying this to processes of (un)becoming a fitness doper, we will focus on what it means to depart from normative models of being young and enter into a subcultural space in which school, work, and other important means of transition into adulthood are put on hold for a certain period of time.

Approaching the Gym

To understand the fitness dopers interviewed and their beginnings at a gym, in this first empirical section of the chapter we focus on their backgrounds and views on training, sport and more. All who have shared their stories currently carry out their principal training at a gym. The amount of time spent on training varies greatly, however. A few participants have been lifting weights since the 1980s, whereas others only have been gym members for a couple of years. Most participants focus on strength training, but there are also some who solely attend group fitness classes or focus on cardio exercise. One commonality in the narratives is that most participants were active in some form of organized sports during adolescence.

The sports movement is by far the most popular recreational activity among children and adolescents in Sweden and many other countries. In addition, there are many indications that various gym training activities have become a significant complement to the exercises organized by traditional sports clubs (Crossley, 2006; Ibsen, 2006; Riksidrottsförbundet, 2011).

Although scholars often have tended to distinguish between training and drug use practices in the sport context and the gym and fitness context, it is obvious that there are clear links between sports associations and the world of gym and fitness, not least in the narratives this book is based upon. The participants have achieved various levels in their respective sports and engaged in a variety of disciplines, but consistently provide information about having been dedicated sportswomen and sportsmen during their youth. Actually, it appears as if their first visit to a fitness facility was often the result of exactly that kind of dedication. Carl explains:

> I started with athletics and such stuff and then it was team handball and badminton. I tried football a few times, but it was, sort of, not my thing. Nah, it was just chasing after the ball. Not much happened. I was hooked on team handball. Then, at the same time I had begun pumping iron a bit. It was in connection with the handball there, because you could become a bit more stable as a 9-meter shot then. And already then, it became clear, not only that you became stronger and all, but that you could withstand blows. (Carl)

For Carl, pumping iron was clearly related to his desire to perform on the team handball court. The logic was simple, by lifting weights he could create a more competitive body. In this sense, his story certainly follows one of organized sports' most basic logics, wanting to train harder to become a better athlete (Guttman, 1978), which also resonates well with the logic of *the athlete type* sketched by Christiansen et al. (2016). Another participant, Stan, has a background in sports that is in many ways reminiscent of Carl's. Stan's introduction to the gym was preceded by high-level junior hockey. Initially, it was Stan's father who urged him to start lifting weights, hoping that he might become more competitive during various clinches on the ice. With his long, thin body, he initially felt out of place in the gym facilities. However, less than a year after his first visit to the gym his experiences of this place had changed considerably. He had grown muscles and wanted to start competing in bodybuilding. Even if this wish was never fulfilled, the strength training came to mean that he would redefine his approach to training and the body. He says:

In the beginning I focused on both hockey and bodybuilding. I thought there were no problems. Then I quit with hockey when I was 18, and then I took the plunge and went for bodybuilding. But when I was 17 and I decided that I would compete, then I was still into hockey. Then, the fact that I quit hockey had probably more to do with the team, I played in a club on the south side of Stockholm, it was more like, they didn't have any first-class teams. Everything just deteriorated. Then I felt that, nah, but then I focused fully on bodybuilding. Then another thing about this, that I liked about the gym, it was that I was there alone, and gave it my all. I didn't have to take lots of other people into account, but hockey's a team sport where you have to take others into account. (Stan)

For Stan, the gym allowed him to further develop not only his body, but also the performance logic he had internalized through his years in organized sport. At the gym, he could challenge himself and monitor the results of his efforts. By gaining knowledge about the body's constitution, developing training strategies and learning to analyze how muscles should be stressed in order to grow, he gradually became his own expert, monitoring his own training. From a Foucauldian perspective, this type of increased self-control and self-monitoring can certainly be seen as an expression of how Stan successively turned his life into a personal work of art (cf. Pedersen, 2010). Furthermore, as a consequence, the muscle-building exercises at the gym and the new ways of perceiving physicality provided Stan with a sense of individual freedom. Because this sense highlights the gap between junior- and senior-level activities in organized sports, it can be linked to fundamental changes in his everyday life and adolescence. The energy and interest previously invested in collective sports activities that were tied to fixed time schedules came to shift over to an increasingly appealing individualistic gym culture that seemed to fit in well with Stan's changing identity claims. Certainly, understood in the light of the emergence of an individualized modern society (Ibsen, 2006), this narrative can be seen as an example of how the individual has come to be held increasingly responsible for shaping his/her own life, through detachment from traditional values and processes of rationalization (Foucault, 1988; Markula & Pringle, 2006).

Thoughts About the Perfect Body

Just as the widely quoted Simone de Beauvoir ([1949] 2010) argued that a woman is something one becomes, not something one is born as, so can the will to change the body through drug use practices be seen as an ongoing endeavor. For Ian's part, it was his desire to become the strongest and best in wrestling that brought him to the gym. He talks about his perspective on the body:

> I've always liked muscles. It has always been a fascination of some kind. Then it was always fun to see how strong you were, how much you could do on the bench press. It was important! (…) You always wanted to be the strongest, huh, for some strange reason. If you're good at something, it becomes more enjoyable, if you notice you're better than everyone else. So that was probably what started it.

Following in the footsteps of bodybuilding giants such as Charles Atlas and Eugen Sandow (Reich, 2010), this description fits perfectly into more stereotypical conceptions of dominant masculinity. However, this fascination with muscles and the body can also be understood as an expression of what Nixon (1996) calls a cultural transformation process, in which men's bodies have become aestheticized and sensualized as pleasurable objects, in a way that has usually been 'reserved for' women's bodies. Actually, this fascination with what one can do with one's body, the creation of muscles, form, symmetry, and more, seems to unite the participants, regardless of gender and whatever body ideal is being pursued.

Another participant, Karin, tells us a little about her fascination with the body and muscles.

> My father was a race horse breeder and I've always been like, really interested in muscled animals. Yes, simply fascinated by muscles. I like it, vital animals and athletic people. So, when I came into the gym when I was 15, I started training a little bit and then felt, this is great fun. Just to have free hands. Bodybuilding is, you sculpt your body. You can decide exactly how you want to look, completely. And I thought that this was a pretty cool experience. I can decide how I look.

The reward system that Karin experienced in the gym environment was different from what she had previously experienced, in sport for example. Attention in the form of lingering glances and encouraging comments caused her training results to connect neatly with her physicality and self-confidence. Her ability to manage and control her body's constitution became an expression of her desire to live a healthy and active life as well as an affirmation of beauty and body ideals. For Karin, like many others, growing muscles and identity in some respects merged to become the same thing.

Young people who spend a great amount of time at the gym gradually become part of a specific group, an inner circle of highly devoted individuals (cf. Lave & Wenger, 1991). These young people develop specific ways of approaching physical culture, the body and the self. Not surprisingly, their preoccupation with training, looks, and bodily esthetics sometimes gets out of control and can lead to a variety of distorted self-images. Marita describes her relation to the body in the following way:

> I've thought about how my body is changing. If you stay away from the fitness center for say a week's time, nothing is actually happening with your body. It's not changing during that short period. But at the same time, you feel something is wrong. It's not the image of yourself you observe in the mirror, it's the image you've created in your mind. It's a feeling. (Marita)

Naturally, such high aspirations and obsession with the ideal body, as exemplified by Marita, are also fueled by media images, the circulation of 'perfect' bodies, and the knowledge and ideology that everything is possible.

In gym and fitness culture, a specific cultural mechanism is developed: *the ideology of the dissatisfied* (Johansson, 1998). Although the participants spend a great deal of time on training and put considerable effort into sculpturing their bodies in the direction of the ideal body, they seem to share the view that their goals cannot be achieved. In many respects, the creation of the perfect or desirable body is seen as a mission impossible. The discrepancy between the lived body and the ideal body does, however, keep the participants on the move, making them try even harder to mold and train the body. This is expressed succinctly by Jeanette:

> The more I exercise, the more I become fixated with my looks. In the beginning I was quite satisfied with my body. But now I just find flaws and defects everywhere. (Jeanette)

This constant striving for the ideal body, as expressed by Jeanette, certainly comes at a high price. The imaginary of the perfect body is closely connected to her routinized, structured way of life. To this end, extreme discipline and a specific way of treating the body permeate her whole life, leading to the development of a specific serious attitude toward herself. This process should largely be understood as a cultural structure found in gym and fitness culture. Naturally, the gradual sliding, expressed as an inclination to see shortcomings rather than advantages, also has an educational impact and can be seen as an essential element of a learning process (Andreasson, 2014). It is part of the knowledge about and gaze directed at fit bodies that Jeanette and others have acquired over time, affecting how she gazes at her own physicality and that of others.

In an attempt to understand various kinds and expressions of over-exercise, a plethora of terms have also been connected to this discussion and used in the literature, such as anorexia athletica, exercise bulimia, and exercise addiction (Manley, O'Brien, & Samuels, 2008). These terms for over-exercise, however, are difficult to define based solely on the amount of exercise. Rather they need to be considered in conjunction with the context in which the exercising occurs, and as a consequence, precise definitions have often been elusive. Naturally, a high frequency of physical training and a strict diet and lifestyle may initially be connected to health, but gradually this 'healthy' lifestyle turns into something different—at times into something quite the opposite of health. Below, Nick tells us about his approach to the gym. Certainly, his way of looking at exercise and the body seems to fit neatly into descriptions of over-exercise and the logic of the dissatisfied.

Nick: You wanted an identity. And it helped after all, when you got muscles. You don't stand out in a regular t-shirt and no muscles. But at the same time, it's hard, sad, and really sad actually. Because you know it never ends.

Jesper: What do you mean sad?

Nick: It's like, I think my body might be made to weigh max 90 kg. And when I weighed 82 kg, I thought I had a damn good body. I could do everything with it, but then I wanted to gain a couple of kilos, thought well I'll go up to 85 then I'll be satisfied. But when you're at 84.5 kilograms, you want to weigh 90. So it turns out completely wrong. You've got to be satisfied at some point. You have to appreciate that enough is enough, now it looks good. But that thought has never presented itself to me. Never.

Aiming for a hard, highly muscular body, Nick has never felt satisfied with his own body. As such, his story and those of others illustrate the thin line and delicate balance between regular training and hard-core dedication, in which PIED use 'suddenly' or gradually becomes an option. For Nick, and many others, gym and fitness exercises are clearly part of a healthy lifestyle, but the gym is also a place where his perception of himself has changed. The paradox is that these temples of the body, the fitness gyms, both harbor body techniques and specialized knowledge that can be used to promote health and contribute to stricter, harsher body ideals and cultivation of the imaginary of the perfect body. The results of this paradox have sometimes been discussed in terms of megarexia, which, in brief, is a distortion of the body image that results in a fear of becoming small and insignificant, or, the opposite, as anorexia nervosa, which usually manifests itself in excessive exercise and self-starvation. Obviously, these medical and psychiatric diagnoses are beyond the scope of this book. Nevertheless, they need to be understood as the effects of specific lifestyle issues, and hence they must be conceptualized in relation to the various social and cultural settings in which they occur (Turner, 2000).

In fitness magazines, we find images of 'perfect bodies,' the message being that the body can be molded, sculpted, and trained into perfection. This is basically the narrative the fitness industry is delivering. On a subjective level, this imaginary and the phantasm of the perfect body are translated into extreme training practices as well as a disciplined lifestyle. This translational process can obviously lead to healthy bodies, but as touched on in this section, there is also a risk that people will be drawn into this fixation on training, the body and its constitution, weight and fat percentages. Although physical exercise helps trim the body and reduce fat, if one is to reach a state of bodily perfection, it also seems necessary to learn everything one can about what to eat and when to eat it. In the next section, we will look more closely at this issue and focus on how our participants have approached PIEDs as a means to achieve these, and other, ambitions.

Approaching Doping

As regards the participants' initial thoughts about and initiation of PIED use, it appears that, for some, using steroids did not cause much concern at all initially. Rather, it was viewed as a 'natural' thing to do, to maintain a desirable pace of physical development and get closer to the goals they had established in their training, say, in conjunction with having reached a plateau. Mick, a dedicated bodybuilder, hardly hesitated before starting to use steroids, which also made the price quite high.

> I was in great shape. I looked great, but I had stepped into this chemical side a bit too much. It became more important than what kind of exercise I did and what diet I had. I let it take over. Because I'm someone who craves knowledge, I devoured it. Then, I tried to go with the chemicals a bit—well a bit too much actually. It became a bit too much for me. (Mick)

As a dedicated young gym-goer, Mick got greedy. He had a well-developed routine and lifestyle plan consisting of diet, training, rest, and supplements. He was impatient, and in his efforts to achieve greater bodily development, he tried taking a 'chemical' shortcut, which resulted in a couple of weeks of hospitalization. Not knowing his physical limitations, the effects of a combination of different supplements, steroids and diuretics placed him in a life-threatening situation that took him months to recover from. Although aware of the seriousness of the situation, Mick did not lose his motivation and dedication. He recognized that he needed a new approach to the drugs, however, and a more balanced relationship between training, doping, and recovery. He came to realize the importance of not only focusing on bodily results, but also familiarizing himself with the different drugs and learning about their side effects.

In one sense, this process could be viewed as a *pharmaceutical self-education* that itself further stimulates the learner's curiosity and desire to know just how much one can achieve with the help of different (illicit) substances. There is no doubt that Mick's narrative highlights the health risks that accompany such curiosity. In another sense, however, the search for knowledge and the process of achieving practical familiarity and becoming a member of a particular subculture suggest that the risk inherent in drug use practices also entails potential benefits in the form of social support. Another participant, Per, talks about how he got involved with fitness doping.

> There was this guy I contacted. He said 'I can fix the stuff for you—you seem so damn serious'. And he said, 'You won't get any results without it.' So, then I got on these Russian Dianabol Steroids, and I had no idea what it was or how I was supposed to take it. But he explained what they would do, and I still lived at home at that time. I was 18, so I had to hide it from my parents and everything. It was something of a gateway or starting point. Suddenly I noticed how things were. And then there were like a lot of these 'ah-a' moments and stuff. Then I understood why these guys who came to the gym in the spring just grew—not incredibly, but they grew and became much stronger, whereas I, who went to the gym all year, was left wondering what the hell I was doing wrong. (Per)

Per had been training seriously for a couple of years when he started thinking about steroids. Initially, however, he did not know enough about the practice. Being a novice, he found a 'master' who supported him and educated him, to some extent. In the process of initiating drug use, he also came to understand and view bodily results from a new angle. He acquired something of a 'doping gaze,' not only toward himself, but also concerning how he came to understand the changing bodies of others. Key in this narrative is also the presence of social support and an inclusive cultural atmosphere.

While the two excerpts above exemplify rather straightforward narratives about doping, others paint a picture of conflicting attitudes and ideals. John says:

> *John:* I remember I was terrified. There was a friend who helped me with this, and he was about to put it (the injection [author's note]) into my leg, and I got a huge steak from the freezer to cool down the entire leg

and a lot of stuff like that. Yes, I was terrified, but I still wanted to get that shit into me.

Jesper: What were you afraid of?

John: That there might be air in the needle, or that it would break. I probably didn't think about the effects of the steroids—it probably wasn't that, nah. It was more the way you did it. And finally, we were in the bathroom for ten minutes and he did it for me and stuff like that. But I didn't do it by myself—it took time before I dared to do it by myself.

Inserting a needle into one's muscle and injecting substances that will help one lift heavier weights, grow, and perform on a higher level is certainly a critical moment in the doping trajectory. Johns' first doping cycle was preceded by a great deal of thinking about whether, and if so how, he should take the drugs. Initially, he felt oral tablets were the best option. In his mind, it was like taking an aspirin for headaches, but with a different pill and for a different 'malady.' As he acquired more knowledge of various drugs and their effects, he concluded that injections would be preferable. He had been told that this method of providing the body with hormones would be 'easier on the body and especially the liver.' At the same time, he felt uneasy using a needle and syringe. Taking the first injection was associated with substance abuse, narcotics, and physical decay—images that were very different from the one he had of himself as a healthy young man with a nice-looking body, living (mostly) in a sound, respectful manner.

This kind of pondering is further exemplified in the quotation below, in which Nick, a former elite-level boxer, tries to describe his process of deciding whether or not to start using doping substances.

I really didn't want to do it. Really, I still thought I got such good development the way it was, and the older guys who went to the gym and competed and stuff—they were on the juice you know, but they always told me 'You shouldn't do it.' It was never that any of them came up and said 'Hey, hey, you want some?' Never. Instead, it was 'Don't do it' (...) So, I thought about it for ages and then I thought 'Nah, I probably will do it.' So a friend and I went off to the neighboring town here and got it, because he wanted to do a course of steroids as well. But even so, I couldn't do it. It wasn't in me to want to stuff myself with that shit. So, I kept on training, and did some boxing, and alternated with that every half year. (...) But this becomes a way of life—once you decide to invest—you have to eat certain foods, at certain times. At that time, we lived together, my girlfriend and I, and it was stressful for her, at least she felt it was. (Nick)

Concerning individuals' commencement of doping, the above excerpt (and the others presented) can be understood on different intersecting levels. *First*, we have the issue of a physical activity background (see also, Andreasson, 2015). Initially, it was Nick's desire to achieve better results in boxing that led him to the gym, and over a five-year period, his interest in boxing decreased while his interest in having a nice-looking body took off.

Second, we have the significance of the social and relational complexities involved in understanding individuals' initiation into doping. For Nick (as well as for John), the social significance of friends in the gym setting is repeatedly touched on in terms of dis-/encouragement, practical social support, and learning about the drugs and how to take them. Nick also brings up his relationship with his former girlfriend. As he gradually became increasingly involved in a strict training routine, he disengaged from his obligations as a partner. Obviously, beginning something implied disengaging from something else—a relationship, a lifestyle, a sense of cultural belonging, etc.

Third, this raises questions concerning how the notion of identity is negotiated in relation to drug use practices. On the one hand, Nick, for example, wanted to be a good partner and family-oriented person. He also wanted to be law-abiding and live a healthy lifestyle. On the other hand, he felt a strong desire to achieve the physical goals he had set for himself. In Nick's case, as well as others,' this resulted both in uncompleted doping courses and in prolonged periods of non-use. Consequently, in such cases the becoming of the fitness doper is to be understood as more complex than a single rite of passage, which also means that caution is necessary when employing theoretical stage models and ideal types to explain drug use practices and trajectories. As heuristic tools, they certainly have some explanatory power. However, there is also a risk that these models, when used to explain fitness doping or even to profile future dopers, will take the analysis and description of different processes leading to doping several steps too far. Further, such models tend to underestimate the sociocultural components involved and how these are embedded in the surrounding society. *Finally*, the excerpts presented here also include strong cultural dimensions/ideals through which processes of legitimization and familiarization are accentuated.

Unbecoming a Fitness Doper

Analyzing drug use practices in gym and fitness culture clearly brings the significance of the body to the fore. Gym and fitness culture is a culture of disciplined bodies. There is a wide range of studies discussing the use of illegal substances from the perspective of doping being a means to accentuate a masculine body and, thus, also a masculine identity project (Andreasson, 2015; Klein, 1993; Liokaftos, 2017; Monaghan, 2001). Although such a perspective is prominent in this chapter as well (and will be further developed in Chapters 7 and 8), it may also be beneficial to add femininity as a factor, when trying to understand fitness doping trajectories and exit processes. Below, Camille explains her perception of steroids and the body:

> I've tried some fat burning pills that count as steroids. /.../ The fact is that men also have some estrogen in their body. If they happen to have a little more than average, unfortunately they can wind up with man-boobs and extra fat in some places. And girls have testosterone. So then I think, like with me—I might happen to have a little more testosterone naturally because I find it easy to become hard and build muscles. And I want to be physically fit but still look like a woman, you know? (Camille)

Camille suggests that steroid use can be understood to exist on a continuum between what is perceived as the 'natural' and 'unnatural' gendered body. The excerpt further clarifies that the use of doping in relation gender is a negotiable issue (McGrath & Chananie-Hill, 2009). Although Camille had used prohibited drugs in an attempt to lose body fat, she has to her knowledge never been the 'object' of suspicion. Attending mainly group fitness activities, she found she was to some extent under the radar of anti-doping campaigns, which she felt were aimed primarily at male bodybuilders. This corresponds with Mogensen's (2011) study, which discussed and critically analyzed Anti-doping Denmark's ways of using degrading images of male bodybuilders to promote a drug-free gym and fitness culture. Focusing on one group of potential users thus appeared to entail the risk of other groups not being considered relevant in anti-doping campaigns. Consequently, in Camille's case, there were other issues that made her stop using prohibited substances to boost her training results. She continues:

> After all, there is this lingering feeling—you feel worried, and it's illegal. You try to operate in the background, so to speak, but you still think about it. I thought about it all the time actually, when I was on: 'What kind of stuff do I have at home?' (Camille)

Another participant continues:

> Someone may knock on your door at any time. You could get dragged out of your bed when sleeping, even if you're a regular person, and all you're doing is going to work…you go home and cook, exercise, eat and sleep. Unfortunately, Sweden's legislation is such that you're not allowed to use steroids, and if you do, you're considered a criminal. Even if you aren't, the law says you are. Living with this, I was concerned about it all the time. (Jeff)

In both Camille's and Jeff's case, the pathway out of doping was preceded by a great deal of serious thinking. Camille did some courses of fat-burning steroids, but her worries about potential encounters with the police made her decide to quit. For Jeff (as well as others interviewed), the situation was similar. He used to compete as a bodybuilder, and on one occasion during a competition, there was drug-testing and the police brought in different contestants for questioning. Jeff left the premises and 'got away,' but the mere thought of what might have happened was enough. He stopped using the drugs for a while and abandoned his dreams of becoming a competitive bodybuilder. Some years later, however, when one of the authors (Jesper) was conducting observations while training, he met up with Jeff, who explained that he had recently initiated a new course of steroids while on a two-week-long vacation in Egypt (where the law is less strict). However, upon returning to Sweden after the vacation, he got thinking about the official policy and perspective in Sweden, which made him quit the initiated course. After that, he felt nervous knowing that the substances would be traceable in his urine for some time.

What this situation illustrates is, *first*, that the transitional process of unbecoming a fitness doper should not necessarily be understood as a demarcated occasion. *Second*, it (once again) highlights the significance of the social, cultural, and national context. Jeff (and others) talks about being viewed with suspicion, by himself and in the eyes of the Other—the state, friends, family, the police, and so on. *Third*, and perhaps implicitly, the excerpts presented above also accentuate the complex relationship between what, in the public discourse, is perceived as extreme expressions of bodybuilding subcultures and the notion of gym and fitness as a mass leisure phenomenon. As suggested by Jeff, on a social level, the idea of bodybuilders is connected to steroid (ab)use and a criminal life, which turns representations of the lifestyle into something grotesque and even deviant (Locks & Richardson, 2012; Mogensen, 2011). At the same time, on a cultural and symbolic level, bodybuilders embody the end-result of extreme dedication to training and diet, which is highly valued within 'mainstream' fitness culture as well (Andreasson & Johansson, 2014).

This complexity—being part of a subculture while aiming for what are perceived as mainstream goals in society—is explicitly touched on in the next excerpt.

> So, I've built myself a home. I have a girlfriend. All that will be gone if I go to jail. Then there's nothing left but a plastic bag with my belongings. Those thoughts made me question my lifestyle. Then I started to think: I have a daughter, and she needs her father. /.../ I chose to quit when I got children. I made that decision then and there. Also, from my point of view, when you deal with this you become very self-centered. You focus on yourself: my meals, my workouts, and if I'm going to make time for cardiovascular training as well. I didn't think it was okay to be like that as a dad. So, I decided to quit. (Hans)

In contrast to the discussion that initiated this section, masculinity (as well as femininity) can form the foundation for unbecoming a user. For Hans, fatherhood and maturity gradually developed into superior masculine ideals, and to this end, unbecoming a fitness doper was largely a matter of leaving a position in which he had pursued muscular masculinity.

Dependency on steroids is tightly interwoven with a specific lifestyle, identity, and body. Quitting these drugs could endanger the person's whole body and lifestyle project. In particular, the fear of losing a certain body and look may have detrimental effects on people's attempts to exit the lifestyle and stop using the drugs. The process of distancing oneself from the cultural context is also touched on in several narratives—for some it was a necessity if they were to unbecome a fitness doper. Included here are also negotiations between different perceptions of an idealized lifestyle. Jim, who still trains on a regular basis but no longer uses PIEDs, explains:

> The training lifestyle—doing bodybuilding—makes it difficult to enjoy life. I mean today, if I'd been okay and not had a cold, I would have gone to the gym after our talk. Yeah, I would go to lift some weights. And then, I'd come home to take a bath and perhaps enjoy a malt whiskey, although I would probably also take a protein shake and some nutrition. But, this feeling of just enjoying life, and having a nice evening, it's unusual for me. Cooking a nice dinner and just enjoying being there. When doing bodybuilding, you have to weigh everything. There are needles here and needles there, pills here and pills there. And then you go off training, and you go powerwalking for two hours in the evening, since you have to keep fit. It's a totally different life. And I mean, it's not so damn healthy. (Jim)

The differences between what is perceived as a 'normal' lifestyle—enjoying good food, social life, and not having to use steroids—and the bodybuilder's life are touched on in several interviews, as in the excerpt above. A common reason for engaging in an exit process—unbecoming a fitness doper and leaving a lifestyle imbued with subcultural values—is the longing for what is perceived to be an ordinary life. As shown, however, the meanings attached to this are various and negotiable.

In this section, we have presented a multitude of reasons why our participants chose to engage in an exit process. As shown, these processes are found on different intersecting levels. *First*, we have the issue of gender and identity, which appears to be relevant when trying to understand doping trajectories. The traditional position in the literature is that muscular masculinities are understood as a trigger for doping, but less researched is how such positions may be contested by other masculine positions, such as that of the responsible father and family man—a topic we will return to in Part III.

Second, this is further accentuated by the particularities of the national and cultural context of use. When doping is prohibited, the risk of potential encounters with the law seems to serve as a reminder, to varying extents, of what could be lost in terms of social relations, marriage, health, freedom, and more. Negotiating the lifestyle-related pros and cons becomes a question of a sense of cultural belonging and identity.

Finally, as argued, our aim is to understand our participants' narratives about their exit processes, and it is difficult to situate them exclusively within a subcultural space. Rather, the cultural mobility exemplified in thought and practice suggests that exit processes need to be understood less as 'either or,' and more as transitional phases. In the next section, we will further develop this discussion, summarizing our thoughts and drawing some conclusions regarding how to theorize about and think through the processes of (un)becoming a fitness doper.

Conclusions

Getting better results, taking 'shortcuts,' and becoming someone desirable are naturally tempting. After crossing what could be described as different barriers, such as injecting steroids into a muscle and contesting the prohibition of the use, the fitness doper gradually invests in subcultural values. However, when we look more closely at doping, it is also obvious that using known 'shortcuts' to achieve desirable results is an idea that is constantly nourished within the more general fitness culture. Kryger Pedersen (2010) describes this tendency as a societal process of *medicalization*. It is a process that, *first*, is characterized by a rationality common in modern medicine, which 'says' that pharmaceuticals provide quick and easy solutions to different physical problems and, therefore, that benefitting from them is logical. *Second*, it is a process that also provides tools for controlling and supervising the health status of the body in transformation. Implicit in this process is a gradual shifting of the individual's perspective on doping, partly disconnecting it from the moralistic, purist, and perhaps romanticized ideals of fair play in modern sport, and connecting it to a scientific and medical discourse (Dimeo & Hunt, 2011).

The exit process is even more complicated. In this process, the fitness doper must unbecome and 'unlearn' and try to enter into what is perceived to be an ordinary life, free from drugs and lofty ambitions. One of the most important driving forces also seems to be the desire to leave a lifestyle that entails criminal activity. The constant risk of being regarded as deviant and criminal creates shame and accentuates the desire to change one's lifestyle. However, this also means re-defining one's sense of self and feelings of belonging. Most importantly, the user is not just leaving a social life—friends, routines, and an entire lifestyle—but also, in fact, a body and carnal experiences. The exit processes are, therefore, seldom straightforward and simple. The linear model described by Ebaugh is a splendid heuristic instrument suitable for looking at sequences, exit processes, and stages. But if we wish to describe the fallacies, the 'hang-over' identity, and the difficulties in adapting to a non-criminal lifestyle, we also need to add discussions based on other theories. In this respect, Halberstam's phenomenology can help us understand the nonlinear and unexpected developments that can occur in the processes of (un)becoming a fitness doper. Taking as our starting point users' own experiences and subjective images of (sub)cultural belonging, we have tried, in this chapter, to highlight the complexity involved in transitional processes of (un)becoming a fitness doper.

Aiming to analytically understand processes of (un)becoming a fitness doper, one obvious commonality found among our participants is their background in organized sport. Traditionally, doping in sports and doping in gym and fitness culture have been researched separately and analyzed as two distinct phenomena. But as indicated in our interviews, this distinction needs to be contested and possibly deconstructed. For example, there is a need for further research on how values and ideals acquired through youth sport participation are transformed when applied/lived in the context of gym and fitness culture. When developing prevention strategies and anti-doping campaigns, the nexus between doping in sport and in society (i.e., in gym and fitness culture) also needs to be taken into consideration.

References

Altier, M. B., Thoroughgood, C. N., & Horgan, J. G. (2014). Turning away from terrorism: Lessons from psychology, sociology, and criminology. *Journal of Peace Research, 51*(5), 647–661.

Andreasson, J. (2014). Shut up and squat: Learning body knowledge within the gym. *Journal of Ethnography and Education, 9*(1), 1–15.

Andreasson, J. (2015). Reconceptualising the gender of fitness doping: Performing and negotiating masculinity through drug-use practices. *Social Sciences, 4,* 546–562.

Andreasson, J., & Johansson, T. (2014). *The global gym: Gender, health and pedagogies.* Basingstoke: Palgrave Macmillan.

Becker, H. S. (1953). Becoming a marihuana user. *American Journal of Sociology, 59*(3), 235–242.

Bell, C., Buono, A., & Rawady, T. (2009). *Bigger stronger faster: The side effects of being American.* Aalborg, Denmark: Sandrew Metronome.

Brennan, R., Wells, J., & Van Hout, M. C. (2017). The injecting use of image and performance-enhancing drugs (IPED) in the general population: A systematic review. *Health and Social Care in the Community, 25*(5), 1459–1531.

Burman, E. (2008). *Deconstructing developmental psychology.* London: Routledge.

Christiansen, A. V. (2009). Doping in fitness and strength training environments—Politics, motives and masculinity. In V. Møller, M. McNamme, & P. Dimeo (Eds.), *EElite sport, doping and public health* (pp. 99–118). Odense: University Press of Southern Denmark.

Christiansen, A. V., Schmidt Vinther, A., & Liokaftos, D. (2016). Outline of a typology of men's use of anabolic androgenic steroids in fitness and strength training environments. *Drugs: Education, prevention and policy.* https://doi.org/10.1080/09687637.2016.1231173.

Crossley, N. (2006). In the gym: Motives, meaning and moral careers. *Body & Society, 12*(3), 23–50.

de Beauvoir, S. (1949/2010). *The second sex.* London: Vintage.

Dimeo, P. (2007). *A history of drug use in sport 1876–1976: Beyond good and evil.* London and New York: Routledge.

Dimeo, P., & Hunt, T. M. (2011). The doping of athletes in the former East Germany: A critical assessment of comparison with Nazi medical experiments. *International Review for Sociology of Sport, 47*(5), 581–593.

DuRant, R., Escobedo, L., & Heath, G. (1995). Anabolic-steroid use, strength training, and multiple drug use among adolescents in the United States. *Pediatrics, 1995*(96), 23–28.

Ebaugh, H. R. F. (1988). *Becoming an ex: The process of role exit.* Chicago: The University of Chicago Press.

European Commission. (2014). *Study on doping prevention: A map of legal, regulatory and prevention practice provisions in EU 28.* Luxembourg: Publications Office of the European Union.

Foucault, M. (1988). *The history of sexuality, vol. 3: The care of the self.* London: Penguin.

Guttman, A. (1978). *From ritual to record: The nature of modern sport.* New York: Columbia University Press.

Halberstam, J. (2005). *In a queer time and place: Transgender bodies, subcultural lives.* New York: New York University Press.

Ibsen, B. (2006). *Foreningsidrætten i Danmark: Udvikling og udfordringar.* Köpenhamn: Idrættens Analyseinstitut.

IHRSA. (2016). *The 2016 IHRSA global report: The state of the health club industry.* Boston: IHRSA.

Johansson, T. (1998). *Den skulpterade kroppen. Gymkultur, friskvård och estetik* [The Sculptured body. Gym culture, wellness and aesthetics]. Stockholm: Carlsson Bokförlag.

Johansson, T. (2017). Youth studies in transition: Theoretical explorations. *International Review of Sociology, 27*(3), 510–524.

Kimegård, A. (2015). A qualitative study of anabolic steroid use amongst gym users in the United Kingdom: Motives, beliefs and experiences. *Journal of Substance Use, 20*(4), 288–294. https://doi.org/10.3109/14659891.2014.911977.

Kimegård, A., & McVeigh, J. (2014). Environments, risk and health harms: A qualitative investigation into the illicit use of anabolic steroids among people using harm reduction services in the UK. *British Medical Journal Open, 2014*(4), 1–7. https://doi.org/10.1136/bmjopen-2014-005275.

Klein, A. (1993). *Little big men: Bodybuilding, subculture and gender construction.* New York: State University of New York Press.

Kryger Pedersen, I. (2010). Doping and the perfect body expert: Social and cultural indicators of performance-enhancing drug use in Danish Gyms. *Sport in Society: Cultures, Commerce, Media, Politics, 13*(3), 503–516.

Lave, J., & Wenger, E. (1991). *Situated learning: Legitimate peripheral participation.* Cambridge: Cambridge University Press.

Liokaftos, D. (2017). *A Genealogy of Male Bodybuilding: From Classical to freaky*. New York and London: Routledge.

Liokaftos, D. (2018). Natural bodybuilding: An account of its emergence and development as competition sport. *International Review for the Sociology of Sport*, 1–18. https://doi.org/10.1177/1012690217751439.

Locks, A., & Richardson, N. (2012). *Critical readings in bodybuilding*. London: Routledge.

Lucidi, F., Zelli, A., Mallia, L., Grano, C., Russo, P., & Violani, C. (2008). The social-cognitive mechanisms regulating adolescents' use of doping substances. *Journal of Sports Sciences, 26*(5), 447–456.

Manley, R., O'Brien, K., & Samuels, S. (2008). Fitness instructors' recognition of eating disorders and attendant ethical/liability issues. *Eating Disorders: The Journal of Treatment and Prevention, 16*(2), 103–116.

Markula, P., & Pringle, R. (2006). *Foucault, sport and exercise: Power, knowledge and transforming the self*. London and New York: Routledge.

McGrath, S., & Chananie-Hill, R. (2009). 'Big Freaky-Looking Women': Normalizing gender transgression through bodybuilding. *Sociology of Sport Journal, 26*, 235–254.

McNamee, M., Backhouse, S. H., Defoort, Y., Parkinson, A., Sauer, M., & Collins, C. (2014). *Study on doping prevention: A map of legal, regulatory and prevention practice provisions in EU 28*. Retrieved from Luxembourg: http://www.studyondopingprevention.eu/.

Mogensen, K. (2011). *Body Punk. En afhandling om mandlige kropsbyggere og kroppens betydninger i lyset av antidoping kampagner* [Body punk. A thesis on male bodybuilders and the meanings of the body in the light of anti-doping campaigns]. Roskilde: Roskilde Universitetscenter.

Monaghan, L. (2001). *Bodybuilding, drugs and risk: Health, risk and society*. New York: Routledge.

Mottram, D. (2005). *Drugs in sport*. London and New York: Routledge.

Nilsson, S., Spak, F., Marklund, B., Baigi, A., & Allebeck, P. (2005). Attitudes and behaviors with regards to androgenic anabolic steroids among male adolescents in a country of Sweden. *Substance Use & Misuse, 40*(1), 1–12.

Nixon, S. (1996). *Hard looks: Masculinities, spectatorship & contemporary consumption*. London: UCL Press.

Reich, J. (2010). "The world's most perfectly developed man": Charles atlas, physical culture, and the inscription of American masculinity. *Men and Masculinities, 12*(4), 444–461.

Riksidrottsförbundet. (2011). *Svenska folkets idrotts- och motionsvanor*. Stockholm: Riksidrottsförbundet.

Sagoe, D., Andreassen, C. S., & Pallesen, S. (2014). The aetiology and trajectory of anabolic-androgenic steroid use initiation: A systematic review and synthesis of qualitative research. *Substance Abuse Treatment, Prevention, and Policy, 9,* 1–14. https://doi.org/10.1186/1747-597x-9-27.

Sassatelli, R. (2010). *Fitness culture: Gyms and the commercialisation of discipline and fun.* Houndmills, UK: Palgrave Macmillan.

Thualagant, N. (2012). The conceptualization of fitness doping and its limitations. *Sport in Society: Cultures, Commerce, Media, Politics, 15*(3), 409–419.

Turner, B. (2000). *Regulating bodies: Essays in medical sociology.* London and New York: Routledge.

Van Hout, M. C., & Hearne, E. (2016). Nethnography of female use of the synthetic growth hormone CJC-1295: Pulses and potions. *Substance Use & Misuse.* https://doi.org/10.3109/10826084.2015.1082595.

Waddington, I. (2000). *Sport, health and drugs: A critical sociological perspective.* London and New York: Routlegde.

Waddington, I., & Smith, A. (2009). *An introduction to drugs in sport: Addicted to winning?* London and New York: Routledge.

Wenger, E. (1998). *Communities of practice.* Cambridge: Cambridge University Press.

Zelli, A., Lucidi, F., & Mallia, L. (2010). The relationships among drive for muscularity, drive for thinness, doping attitudes, and doping intentions in adolescents. *Journal of Clinical Sport Psychology, 4*(1), 39–52.

6

Fitness Doping Online

Introduction

Internationally, governments and public health organizations are conducting fairly comprehensive anti-doping campaigns (Locks & Richardson, 2012; Mogensen, 2011). This development, combined with the technological developments of recent decades, has resulted in the emergence of other ways of learning about and accessing performance- and image-enhancing drugs (PIEDs). For instance, social media and Internet forums have become part of a new self-help culture in which people can anonymously approach PIEDs, discuss their experiences, and at the same time minimize the risk of legal repercussions (Hsiung, 2000; Monaghan, 2012).

Obviously, online forums and communities encourage posting of sensitive content without compromising confidentiality and facilitate long-term in-depth discussions (Smith & Stewart, 2012). Online communities may also be particularly attractive, as they facilitate access to information and discussions that are normally hidden from the general public and the authorities (Saba & McCormick, 2001). This has been shown in several studies (see, e.g., Adler & Adler, 2005, 2011; Lynch, 2010; Monaghan, 2012). For example, Smith and Stewart (2012) conducted a study on an

© The Author(s) 2020
J. Andreasson and T. Johansson, *Fitness Doping*,
https://doi.org/10.1007/978-3-030-22105-8_6

online bodybuilding community hosted in the USA, showing how this community appears to strengthen the self-perception of its members, on the one hand, while the drug use promoted in the community sometimes leads to identity conflicts and self-doubt, on the other. Common to these studies is that, in different ways and to different extents, they raise the question of how online communications and online identity constructions can help users become aware of and learn more about particular practices.

This chapter focuses on how the use of PIEDs is perceived and negotiated socially in the context of one open online community: Flashback. This community describes itself as Sweden's largest forum for freedom of expression, opinion, and independent thinking (Flashback, n.d.), and may therefore be considered a highly open-minded forum as regards prohibited activities such as PIED use. We are interested in how such use is discussed on Flashback and how participants begin coming closer to and learning about this practice in the community. By analyzing how Flashback members approach PIEDs and discuss these drugs' effects, we first suggest that it is possible to capture the gradual process through which the practice gradually transforms or influences users' perception of body and self. Second, we suggest that it is possible to connect these narratives to the creation of a certain doping trajectory situated within fitness culture.

Community of Practice and Drug Use

Using a constructionist approach (Berger & Luckmann, 1966; Hacking, 2000), in this chapter we look at how particular subject positions (identities) and drug use strategies evolve within a specific online community, which is understood as a kind of 'community of practice' (CofP): Here, a CofP is understood as:

> An aggregate of people who come together around mutual engagement in an endeavour. Ways of doing things, ways of talking, beliefs, values, power relations – in short, practices – emerge in the course of this mutual endeavour. As a social construct, a CofP is different from the traditional community, primarily because it is defined simultaneously by its membership and by the

practice in which that membership engages. (Eckert & McConnell-Ginet, 1992, p. 464)

Joining an Internet community inevitably involves aspects of both learning and identity construction (Lave & Wenger, 1991; Wenger, 1998). For example, learning processes regarding drug use and the physical experiences resulting from this practice are intersubjective (Becker, 1953). The inclination to engage in PIED use is seen as something the individual acquires during the process of learning, through communication with others, about the actual activity, resulting in changes in users' perception of the activity. Consequently, the learning process involved in becoming a PIED user is not only intersubjective in nature, but also transformative, meaning that the experience of drug use practices varies within the individual over time and space, as he/she learns about how to understand and experience the practice. Put differently, when people decide to join an online community and perhaps also to use PIEDs in their training, they learn from others' experience, which changes their conception of the practice and, consequently, their understanding of themselves, what they can do, and how they perceive others (Andreasson, 2014; Monaghan, 2001a). The ways in which people use and understand their bodies are an expression of the integration of learning processes and the ongoing process of continuous identity performance and construction (Biesta, 2006). Similar processes and identity formations are also present in subcultures. It is, therefore, also possible to discuss PIED use narratives found in online communication in relation to subcultural affiliations.

As individuals gain experience and articulate and discuss theories about how to reach their desired goals, they also become increasingly involved in a particular Internet community. Some people in the community will choose to take drugs, and by doing so deviate from certain norms and values in mainstream society. Others in the community will do their best to stay within the bounds of the prevailing societal order. An Internet community or subculture does not assume role homogeneity, but rather focuses on the ways in which people speak about and engage in different kinds of practices. Consequently, on the one hand, within a specific subculture, members must adopt appropriate behaviors, symbolically at least, in order to function (Smith & Stewart, 2012). On the other hand, the nature of online interaction enables members to make their 'virtual identity' independent of their physical one, at least to some extent. In our understanding of the concept of identity in the context of online communities, we have been inspired by Turkle (1995), who suggests that the use of Internet communications creates not only opportunities to perform an alternative identity, but also the basis for an alternative lifestyle. In this respect, we interpret the concept of identity in a multidimensional fashion. We suggest that the narratives presented should be understood as markers of identity, but we also recognize that, due to their pseudo-anonymity, participants may assume a contrived identity, perhaps one that will result in social recognition and status within the community (Giles, 2006).

The process of learning how to become a PIED user is inevitably interwoven with a larger system of relationships with others, such as gym owners, lawmakers, media reporters and, of course, Internet contacts (Sassatelli, 2010). Hence, the becoming and education of a PIED user entail the individual becoming part of a process through which relationships are reshaped, which provides new opportunities and enables the individual to assume new positions in the larger relational systems in which he/she participates. In a *subcultural space* such as the one studied in this chapter and touched on in Chapter 5, the goal of transforming the body into something else, something perfect, could take precedence over other goals. In this process of transforming the body through PIED use, the distinctions between safe and unsafe, legal and illegal, healthy and sick, as well as shameless and shameful can be partially destabilized or renegotiated. One of the ambitions of this chapter is to analyze the ways in which the individual learns how to transform the self through drug use and the ways in which this practice is rationalized within a specific online community.

Resisting the Law

The reasons for joining an Internet community certainly may differ. Logically, membership is preceded by curiosity about the particular activity being discussed by other members. On Flashback, there are many people who seem to be novices and who express a desire to learn, asking for advice about using PIEDs. When answering such questions, in contrast to the supportive attitudes often expressed by other members of the community, Swedish official policy on and public attitudes toward PIEDs are colored by distrust and dislike. PIED use is often associated with crime and abuse of other drugs; it is described in terms of deviance (DuRant, Escobedo, & Heath, 1995; Moberg & Hermansson, 2006; Skarberg & Engström, 2007). As stated earlier, not only is possession of doping substances prohibited in Sweden, but also the presence of these substances in the body (Kryger Pedersen, 2010). As PIEDs can usually be traced in the human body for quite some time, depending on the substance involved, the decision to begin using also entails possible encounters with the authorities (Christiansen & Bojsen-Møller, 2012). This issue is broadly called into question on Flashback.

> Why do the police want to stop us? There's something fishy going on. That's clear. Results that you could get from AAS within a year now take 3–5 years instead. Why? Is it a conspiracy against ripped guys? There aren't many people who have the patience to get there, and if there were a shortcut, surely loads of people would train to get in shape. (NoPolice)

In the above thread and subsequent postings by other members, there is a certain degree of understanding for the legislation banning PIEDs, or as they are called above, anabolic–androgenic steroids (AAS). Opinions supporting the legislation revolve mainly around the potential side effects of PIEDs as well as the societal costs such substances may entail. These arguments, however, are usually countered with postings in which prohibition is questioned, as in the posting quoted above, and explained as the result of, say, 'media propaganda,' the decision-making of 'ignorant politicians,' or the 'envy' of ordinary people. Responses like these can be compared to what Sykes and Matza (1957) call 'techniques of neutralization,' here meaning that community members try to shift the focus of attention and deflect the negative sanctions attached to PIED use by condemning the condemners. Another member continues the discussion on Swedish law and policy.

> Regarding doping substances, I think that Swedish government policy is idiotic. Certainly it's true that many people commit violent crimes due to

steroid use, but on the other hand there are also many who manage their bodybuilding hobby in an exemplary fashion. Doping should clearly be legal (I'm talking about hobby doping; obviously I don't defend cheating in competitions). The doping ban is a consequence of the government's feministic hatred of men. Smash the state! (Legalise)

Clearly, there is not much identification with a political agenda of gender equality built into this posting. This understanding of the practice is also detached from how it may be used in organized sport in order to cheat; it is instead connected to a more neoliberal, individualistic ideology. In a similar way, Monaghan (2012), who both studied pro-steroid Internet bodybuilding forums and ethnographically followed PIED users, shows that one of the strategies used to justify fitness doping is to promote condemnation of what is thought to be other people's unfounded and unreflective criticism. Although some of the threads deal with the contradictory emotions involved in this activity, using steroids is not significantly problematized here. Instead, the discussions seem to be primarily characterized by a pragmatic approach and perspective, and therefore, tend to reduce the effectiveness of the social control represented by the authorities. In this way, the learning about the trade and the trajectory to drug use follows a familiar path found in the literature on deviant careers (see, e.g., Becker, 1953; Monaghan, 2012; Myers, 1992). First, community members formulate arguments claiming that the threats posed by authorities are limited (like above); second, as below, interdependence is created between members to ensure that supplies can be distributed.

In the following posting, one community member presents a checklist showing how to remain invisible to the police.

We start with the bank transfer. Do not use your Internet bank. If your providers get caught and the police go through their accounts, they'll easily find your transaction. [...] Ok, so the question is how to send money. By mail. Preferably use a padded envelope. Fold the money in something before placing it in the envelope – for example, stiff paper or foil or the like, so that no one can see what the envelope contains. (Mailman)

These instructions are followed by hundreds of related postings. This would seem to be a theme that many members find relevant. After giving step-by-step instructions regarding where and how to order and how to pay, Mailman presents a checklist containing several points. For example, readers are instructed to use encrypted e-mail, to constantly delete e-mail correspondences, to erase notes containing names, and to throw away post office receipts. Altogether, this thread amasses some fairly comprehensive instructional content on how to behave when dealing with steroids on the Internet and how to minimize the risk of legal repercussions. In this way, new members are gradually guided into the subcultural space and supported through the different and mostly encouraging arguments, considerations, and attitudes displayed adjacent to the instructions.

What is taking place here is social diffusion of knowledge, through which the legislation prohibiting PIEDs is questioned and the individual's curiosity is heightened. Consequently, within a specific community, like the one analyzed in this chapter, members find ways to justify and rationalize their practice. The trajectory leading to PIED use starts when the individual learns about the practice and becomes interested and willing to engage in the activity (cf. Becker, 1953). In the Flashback community, members find support in constructing an understanding of the practice, which in this case serves to challenge the logic of the Swedish legislation. Thus, in this process, it is not only physiological boundaries that are challenged through actual or intended drug use, but also the social control exerted by the Swedish state through legislation.

This first empirical section of the chapter provides a preview of the attitudes, strategies, and ethos that develop in this particular kind of Internet community. In the next two sections, we look more closely at how Flashback members develop their arguments, and consequently, their understanding of how to talk about, relate to, and use PIEDs. We focus particularly on how community members develop their self-understanding and identity in relation to the social diffusion of knowledge about PIEDs.

Transcending Identities and Potential Health Risk

There are many studies focusing on people's attempts to attain the 'perfect' body using legal or illegal means (Monaghan, 1999b; Thualagant, 2012).

In an ethnographic study, Atkinson (2007) showed how young men used different kinds of legal supplements not only to control their bodies, but also to gain social recognition as part of a more general self-presentation. In the story below, a community member describes the first time he used a PIED and in so doing provides an illustration of how use of prohibited substances can be related to self-understanding.

> So after much consideration, it's finally time to take the plunge, take the final step, and run a course (of steroids) to see what it can bring. I've been wanting to do this since I started going to the gym, but for various reasons always changed my mind at the last minute. Now that I'm older, I've got a little more meat on my bones and have learned how to acquire knowledge and make my own decisions. So I've decided to run a course of Dianabol, which seems to suit my goals best. Whether this is true or not, time will tell. […] Below, I will sum up the first week and as briefly as possible describe my progress and my thoughts about the experience. Initially I didn't plan to write a report but then I thought it might be kind of therapeutic, and might also encourage others to give me good advice. (MeatOnBone)

This description can be read as indicating an ongoing construction of feelings, expectations, and attitudes and, as such, is a marker of identity. The poster's use of the handle MeatOnBone describes the outcome of his first experience of steroids in detail. On the seventh day of the drug regime, readers learn that, following a back session, MeatOnBone 'got so pumped up on my lats I almost thought I could fly.' This empowering narrative is constructed in such a way that it can be used to establish the course for future accomplishments and physical results. At the same time, however, the narrative also contains descriptions of various side effects, such as headaches, dizziness, and nausea, and periodically a constant erection, resulting in the 'need to jerk off at least a couple times a day.' Despite the seriousness of these unwanted side effects, MeatOnBone did not lose his motivation or dedication. Rather, he used Flashback to discuss his experiences. Consequently, MeatOnBone expresses his awareness of some of the risks inherent in PIED use practice. At the same time, his knowledge seeking, the process of 'practical familiarities' and being a member of this subcultural space seem to function as a kind of reassurance that keeps such worries at bay.

In addition, there are situations when the risks of the drug regime present themselves in unexpected ways. For example, when MeatOnBone's body quickly responded to the drug regime, a fellow employee at work confronted him with questions regarding PIED use. Initially he felt proud, but then he became worried, realizing that the questions were reproachful rather than encouraging. In one posting, he says he denied having anything to do with PIEDs and made up a story about his new workout routine and diet. In response to this comment, other community members posted supportive comments, offering alternative inspirational arguments that could be used in similar situations. It is, thus, not only the fear of getting caught breaking the law that is implicitly being negotiated here, but also the potential shame of taking a shortcut in one's quest for desired results. Consequently, in the supportive context of the community, it becomes obvious how pride in one's own physical transformation can rapidly turn into shame about one's body (Sparkes, Batey, & Owen, 2012). This shows how potential pride in and shame about oneself and one's body are clearly to be viewed as interdependent. The following excerpt further develops the theme of the limit-pushing potential of PIEDs in relation to users' regular jobs.

I'm about to start this thread because I'm incredibly fascinated by the effects that steroids have on the human psyche. I would like to hear about other users' experiences and how steroids have affected their working lives. For example, say you're an ordinary employee at a company. Coincidentally, after your first course of steroids, you want to advance to a management position and you succeed in doing so. Or you're a student who experiences a change in your academic performance from mediocre to highly motivated and higher achieving. You see where I'm going with this thread. AAS is so much more than bulky muscles. (HighAchiever)

The comments on this thread, which number in the hundreds, describe a process of transformation, mainly based on adjectives that describe how the self becomes more of something: more ambitious, motivated, aggressive, focused, and attractive. Development of these qualities is frequently described in positive terms, but occasionally mentioned are negative consequences, such as getting into fights. Nevertheless, it is obvious that, in this context, PIED use works as a powerful symbol of an expected transformation and construction of the body and the self. It is a symbol of what could be described as a rite of passage (Gennep, 2004). Below, a Flashback community member describes the expectations generated by using PIEDs. Here, the first injection is seen as something of a milestone, marking an important and decisive stage in a physical transition. The heading of the thread is 'No Guts, No Glory.'

> My first injection accomplished. Start gentle. My opinion is that you should not accelerate like an idiot the first time you try a new and unfamiliar vehicle! The virgin cost me two needles and an office chair, but I have now faced fucking 500 mg of Testo C! Mission accomplished! It's time to get real! Be great or be nothing! I am so fucking powered up now. It will surely be interesting to see how things turn out at the gym. While working out clean, I have already managed to increase the number of reps on some exercises, despite my diet, so there will probably be like a swelling explosion with the juice in my system! (FirstInjection)

FirstInjection's narrative of his rite of passage is clearly dominated by dramatic expectation, confidence, and the imagery of explosively bursting through his bodily limits. It also contains aspects of fear and the need to manage risk, such as when the reader learns that the first needle broke when, during the injection, FirstInjection passed out and fell out of his chair. This did not stop FirstInjection, however, so when he came to, the anticipated rapid effect of the PIED still felt appealing enough. On the second try, the drugs were successfully injected into his thigh.

An approach in which the PIED is viewed as something of a miracle cure, expected to give visible results in a matter of days, is expressed in several threads. Usually, an apparent novice asks others for advice regarding how to organize a drug course. In the posting below, one participant answers another member's question regarding the potential risks and health costs involved in drug use practices. The question posed is: 'How dangerous are steroids, and could you die?'

> Answer: One thing is that you're supposed to not overdo it and dribble too much with doses. The risks are far higher then. For a while I was completely wild, and mixed loads of different steroids. Today I only do *testo*, that's all,

and I feel pretty good about it. The only thing I'm not so happy about is the hair on my back and a few other things. (Don'tOverdo)

The above excerpt provides significant clues about how the process of learning to be a PIED user may be manifested as a personal doping trajectory. The user Don'tOverdo used to go 'wild,' but has learned, through experience, how to run courses in a safer and more controlled manner and still get results. Don'tOverdo then continues the posting by presenting a complete chart over the personal course of treatment he followed. Thus, Don'tOverdo assumes the role of the teacher, explaining to the novice how to proceed and what to expect. In addition, in the same thread there are postings by other members mentioning side effects such as acne, 'bitch tits' (gynecomastia), and even death as possible costs to one's health associated with poorly managed PIED use. Many of these postings also offer advice on how to recognize signs of risk and how to deal with unwanted side effects, should they occur. In some of these discussions, considerable attention is paid to particular substances and what to expect with various types of steroids.

> I don't want to go on any mega bulk. I just want to try and see what happens, and what I want to test is Wintablets (Winstrol). Anyway, this is my first posting here as well. I did some research on where to get the stuff, but I haven't found anything 'new'. So I was wondering where I can get it? I'd also like to know what course you guys would recommend. (Wintab)

> Answer: I have never taken wins (Winstrol), but it's definitely something I want to try when I get a little more weight on. But I have a friend who chewed wins – good stuff. Otherwise, you could take a course of Anavar. You can buy wins from Madman – a quick and green supplier. Always maintain a good standard! (GoodStuff)

In the Flashback community, there are many threads discussing a variety of steroids and offering various opinions on bodily ambitions and pursued goals. In this way, the choice of a particular drug also becomes an expression of identity. If you want to have a supple, vascular body, certain steroids are said to be suitable, whereas if you want to build up mass and gain weight, others might be more appropriate. Monaghan (2002) suggests that this increasing experimentation with different substances—supplements and drugs—is part of the *new ethno-pharmacology* that has become entrenched and ritualized in gym and fitness culture. This bodybuilding-related ethno-pharmacological stock of knowledge is discernable within bodybuilding subculture and comprises: a taxonomy of different steroids, theories of usage, methods of administration, and awareness of effects, possible side effects, and strategies to avoid or attenuate these side effects (Monaghan, 2012, p. 80). As an example of this ethno-pharmacology, many postings we analyzed also seemed to imply that experienced bodybuilders should be understood as being more educated on PIED use than physicians are. Monaghan (1999a) also suggests that bodybuilding, perhaps more than any other athletic pursuit, takes place in a sociocultural environment that normalizes the instrumental use of steroids. In striving to create the perfect body, many muscle enthusiasts view taking drugs as a legitimate means of attaining a subculturally prescribed goal (Monaghan, 1999a). It is important to keep in mind, however, that although the individuals who give others advice on Flashback appear to be relatively knowledgeable and well informed, information regarding where and how these people obtained their knowledge is limited. The ideas that develop in this subcultural space can therefore be understood as a mixture of medical pronouncements and expertise, ethno-scientific knowledge, personal experience, and lay theories of how to achieve the perfect body, as it is expressed by members. Deciding whose advice to follow in the postings can thus involve a hazardous game of negotiating and managing the risks inherent in this scenario.

In sum, on Flashback there are basically no limits as to what subjects may be discussed, and steroids are widely promoted as part of a new self-help culture of ethno-pharmacology (see also, Berns, 2011; Monaghan, 2012). As such, use of different steroids can be seen as constructed within a neoliberal, do-it-yourself method of 'getting fit' or becoming 'healthy,' as a means of attaining social authority and, of course, as a way to ensure continuous bodily development at the gym (Atkinson, 2007; Glasner, 1990). Furthermore, by discussing and developing theories of how to set up different courses, the practice can also be constructed as being performed in the context of a health promoting agenda (Monaghan, 1999a).

Steroids and the Genetic Maximum

The global community that is fitness and bodybuilding culture has developed its own symbolic language and way of talking about different aspects of this form of physical culture. One term often used in relation to taking steroids to boost muscles is the 'genetic maximum' or the 'genetic max.'

The relationship between steroids and a person's genetic max is complex. Steroids are often used to exceed one's genetic max, but sometimes the talk concerns how to use steroids to reach that 'max.' Conceptual discussions about the genetic max can consequently be understood as a mixture of conceptions of physical potential and (sometimes dramatic) fantasies about what is humanly possible to achieve (Locks & Richardson, 2012). Most participants in this culture/context would probably agree that it is almost impossible to determine a person's genetic max. Basically, most members agree that steroids improve results and help increase the muscle builder's body mass.

> Steroids are a shortcut to fast development of muscle mass and strength. Results can be achieved in a short time. But how difficult is it to maintain these results? Now we're not referring to IFBB builders on 120 kilos, who will of course lose muscle mass quickly if they stop using steroids /.../ However, when a man decides to stop using the drugs, but continues to exercise frequently and intensively, will he be able to keep his muscle mass and strength while staying clean? (StillMuscular?)

> Answer: If we're talking about a single cure, it's easy. The closer you are to your potential, the harder it'll be. If you've added 15 kilo of quality muscle (not fluid) you'll have to work hard, but it's not totally impossible. (HardWork)

Many of the comments in this thread on how to maintain muscle mass without using steroids are pessimistic regarding the possibility to remain 'clean' and preserve a given muscle mass and strength. Building muscles without steroids is often described using terms such as stagnation, regression, and futility. Below, one member reflects on what happens when someone gets clean.

I believe you lose more than your imagine. As for me, I'm far above my genetic max. The effects of stopping steroids will be remarkable. The last time I lost a lot of my body mass in just the first two weeks. If I go off the steroids, I'll probably look the same as I did before starting with AAS, because at that time I had already reached my genetic maximum. (GoBefore)

For many practitioners, the goal is not to become yourself and strengthen your 'old' identity, but rather to become someone else, and possibly exceed your genetic maximum. Developing and nourishing this perspective also accommodates the inherent difficulty of disengaging with drug use practices, as it suggests a return to your previous identity, an identity you left behind. Naturally, the anticipated effects of PIEDs and the process of transformation are also largely connected to the issue of gender and most often to the construction of a dominant, muscular, and self-assured masculinity (Denham, 2008; also see Chapter 7).

Even though most participants in the discussion are engaged in a quest to find ways to increase their body mass and strength, there is also a certain awareness of the problematic side of this quest. This is expressed in the form of counter-ideals, discussions about people who have succeeded in keeping themselves clean. While most of these discussions end up describing defeat, thus affirming the importance of steroids, there are exceptions.

Here's a guy who's clean: Aaron Curtis. He only participates in the natural bodybuilding competitions. He has really good sponsors, because he's clean. He has 250,000 followers on Facebook. Check him out. He seems to be an honest person, seems to have good self-knowledge, and also shows extreme self-discipline. (Natural)

Aaron Curtis is a relatively well-known name in bodybuilding circles, particularly through his aim of becoming the best natural bodybuilder he possibly can. Regarding the use of PIEDs, Curtis is quite reproachful. On his Facebook page, he states: 'In my opinion, people should have to earn the right to enhance, not just use performance-enhancing drugs as short-cuts to a physique that could have been attained naturally if they had just learned the basics first.' On Flashback and other bodybuilding sites, there is an ongoing discussion about how 'natural' Aaron Curtis's body really is and if it is possible to reach body goals without drugs.

On Flashback, there seems to be a need for stories affirming that steroid use is a completely sound and rational practice. There is also a constant demand for new ways of transforming and sculpting the body to perfection. Body enhancement drugs are intrinsic to this online culture, and there are even people who speculate about how one can influence and change the basic prerequisites of the human physical form. In this regard, we are witnessing the development of ideas about scientifically engineered 'cyborg bodies' (Pitts, 2003). The following comment speculates on the consequences of this development, which is partly understood as a process of approaching science fiction and 'space facts.'

> So, genetic max? Maybe it *is* possible to influence and improve on your genetic max. People using growth hormones, who let their body grow (the skeleton and the number of muscle cells), also have to influence and change their genetic max, I guess. Or is this just about how much testosterone the body is producing? Cause, I've heard that, if you reach your genetic max, and start using growth hormones to increase your muscle cells and skeleton you can push your genetic max forward and reach another limit. After doing this, you can start to build 'clean.' This is maybe just 'space facts,' I don't know. (Rejman)

Young men and women building their bodies seem to be looking for different ways of enhancing volume and strength. Even though the claims made by, for example, Curtis indicate that it should be possible to reach one's goals in 'natural ways,' most practitioners seem to be convinced that this is more or less an illusion. Therefore, although the above excerpts indicate a certain trend toward natural bodybuilding, there seems to be no easy way out of the shortcut that PIED use represents.

Conclusions

This chapter has hopefully given readers insight into some of the characteristic dynamics of a symbolic community, and into how the relationship between bodies, self-understanding, and PIEDs is discussed in the online community Flashback. We have gained access to what can be considered an extreme sociocultural reality, defined by an intense interest in muscular development and size. In this respect, our results are in line with findings from similar studies on Internet bodybuilding communities (see, e.g., Smith & Stewart, 2012). Although the participants are to some degree aware of the risks and health costs of this kind of bodily regime, the potential benefits of using PIEDs clearly dominate the discussions (see also Monaghan, 2001b).

Reading different postings on Flashback takes us into a specific symbolic and social community. A particular language game is developed, and the discussions about PIEDs often incorporate esoteric ethnomedical terminology. Nutrition, supplements, training regimes, and PIEDs are all part of a highly rationalized, means-to-an-end lifestyle within the subculture. Here, pushing one's physical limits and creating an impressively muscular body is seen as a core value and part of a successful self-presentation.

In the community, ideas circulate about the genetic max, as well as the ultimate possibility of exceeding one's limits and creating something beautiful, special, and extraordinary. The stories on Flashback often affirm the legitimacy of striving for the perfect bodybuilding adventure, as well as the perfect body, using any and all means and methods necessary to mold the ultimate strong body. The 'natural' and 'clean' bodybuilder is constructed as the product of a moral fantasy, and attempts to promote this approach to bodybuilding are opposed by most of the postings found in this subcultural space. In this particular culture, the master or teacher is not a 'natural bodybuilder,' but rather a person who seems prepared to acquire and use all available knowledge to construct the perfect body. This does not imply, however, that a universal representation of a specific physicality is being idealized in the community (Monaghan, 1999b). There are heterogeneous body projects and diverse ways of creating a personalized picture of the perfect body.

The main finding in this chapter is that the online community contributes to specific learning processes. Looking at this as a rite of passage helps us discern how different relations between 'teachers' and 'pupils' are developed, how expert knowledge is diffused and transferred, and how personal doping trajectories gradually develop over time. For example, the first injection is seen as a milestone. The community members function as advisers and supporters of the individual's transformational identity processes. These learning processes include detailed advice on both how to understand and use PIEDs and how to manage risk. Subsequently, these processes also involve a reflexive attitude toward PIED use. Learning how to become a user involves a certain degree of risk-taking and a willingness to use various means to obtain the idealized body, as well as the acquisition of ethno-scientific knowledge that the user can employ to construct the practice as something being performed within a health promoting agenda.

The Internet community under study—Flashback—can be viewed as an example of a community that promotes a transformational process through which ordinary rules and regulations are questioned and put out of play. What we are studying here is a process of deregulation and de-normalization that increases the acceptance of certain kinds of drug use. This process of normalization and acceptance of drug use within the community is in accordance with neoliberal attitudes and the cult of the individual, making it possible to transgress and challenge norms and regulations (see also Miller & Rose, 2008). These processes are of course connected to a general discussion concerning how neoliberal discourses have penetrated our thinking about individual freedom and health (Rich & Evans, 2013). Certainly, the gym and fitness industry, and the practices carried out in these contexts, fit nicely into a neoliberal world view, where people are considered individually responsible for their own body and health. In some ways, striving to achieve the perfect body even makes it logically necessary to challenge legislation on PIEDs and to develop subcultural norms and values. And in the Internet community studied in this chapter, people have access to a great deal of knowledge and find substantial support for the notion that they need to use certain means, and illicit drugs, to achieve their goals.

References

Adler, P., & Adler, P. (2005). Self-injurers as loners: The social organization of solitary deviance. *Deviant Behavior, 26*(4), 345–378.
Adler, P., & Adler, P. (2011). The cyber worlds of self-injurers: Deviant communities, relationships, and selves. *Symbolic Interaction, 31*(1), 33–56.

Andreasson, J. (2014). Shut up and squat. Learning body knowledge within the gym. *Journal of Ethnography and Education, 9*(1), 1–15.

Atkinson, M. (2007). Playing with fire: Masculinity, health and sports supplements. *Sociology of Sport Journal, 24,* 165–186.

Becker, H. S. (1953). Becoming a marihuana user. *American Journal of Sociology, 59*(3), 235–242.

Berger, P. L., & Luckmann, T. (1966). *The social construction of reality: A treatise in the sociology of knowledge.* Garden City, NY: Anchor Books.

Berns, N. (2011). *Closure: The rush to end grief and what it costs us.* Philadelphia: Temple University Press.

Biesta, G. (2006). *Beyond learning: Democratic education for a human future.* Boulder, CO: Paradigm Publishers.

Christiansen, A. V., & Bojsen-Møller, J. (2012). Will steroids kill me if I use them once? A qualitative analysis of inquiries submitted to the Danish anti-doping authorities. *Performance Enhancement & Health, 1,* 39–47.

Denham, B. E. (2008). Masculinities in hardcore bodybuilding. *Men and Masculinities, 11*(2), 234–242.

DuRant, R., Escobedo, L., & Heath, G. (1995). Anabolic-steroid use, strength training, and multiple drug use among adolescents in the United States. *Pediatrics, 96,* 23–29.

Eckert, P., & McConnell-Ginet, S. (1992). Think practically and look locally: Language and gender as community-based practice. *Annual Review of Anthropology, 21,* 461–490.

Flashback. (n.d). *Flashback forum.* Retrieved from https://www.flashback.org/.

Gennep, A. V. (2004). *The rites of passage* (1st ed., 1960). London: Routledge.

Giles, D. C. (2006). Constructing identities in cyberspace: The case of eating disorders. *British Journal of Social Psychology, 45,* 463–477.

Glasner, B. (1990). Fit for postmodern selfhood. In H. S. Becker & M. M. McCall (Eds.), *Symbolic interaction and cultural studies* (pp. 215–243). Chicago: University of Chicago Press.

Hacking, I. (2000). *The social construction of what?.* Cambridge: Harvard University Press.

Hsiung, R. C. (2000). The best of both worlds: An online self-help group hosted by a mental health professional. *Cyber Psychology & Behavior, 3*(6), 935–950.

Kryger Pedersen, I. (2010). Doping and the perfect body expert: Social and cultural indicators of performance-enhancing drug use in Danish gyms. *Sport in Society: Cultures, Commerce, Media, Politics, 13*(3), 503–516.

Lave, J., & Wenger, E. (1991). *Situated learning: Legitimate peripheral participation.* Cambridge: Cambridge University Press.

Locks, A., & Richardson, N. (Eds.). (2012). *Critical readings in bodybuilding.* New York: Routledge.

Lynch, M. (2010). From food to fuel: Perceptions of exercise and food in a community of food bloggers. *Health Education Journal, 71*(1), 72–79.

Miller, P., & Rose, N. (2008). *Governing the present: Administering economic, social and personal life.* Cambridge: Polity Press.

Moberg, T., & Hermansson, G. (2006). *Mandom, mod och morske män* [Manhood, courage and fearless men]. Mölnlycke: Mediahuset.

Mogensen, K. (2011). *Body punk: En afhandling om mandlige kropbyggere og kroppens betydninger i lyset af antidoping kampagner* [Body punk: A thesis on male bodybuilders and the meanings of the body in the light of anti-doping campaigns]. Roskilde: Roskilde Universitetscenter.

Monaghan, L. F. (1999a). Challenging medicine? Bodybuilding, drugs and risk. *Sociology of Health & Illness, 21*(6), 707–734.

Monaghan, L. F. (1999b). Creating 'the perfect body': A variable project. *Body & Society, 5,* 267–290.

Monaghan, L. F. (2001a). *Bodybuilding, drugs and risk: Health, risk and society.* New York: Routledge.

Monaghan, L. F. (2001b). Looking good, feeling good: The embodied pleasures of vibrant physicality. *Sociology of Health & Illness, 23*(3), 330–356.

Monaghan, L. F. (2002). Vocabularies of motive for illicit steroid use among bodybuilders. *Social Science and Medicine, 55,* 695–708.

Monaghan, L. F. (2012). Accounting for illicit steroid use: Bodybuilders' justifications. In A. Locks & N. Richardson (Eds.), *Critical readings in bodybuilding.* New York: Routledge.

Myers, J. (1992). Nonmainstream body modification: Genital piercing, branding, burning, and cutting. *Journal of Contemporary Ethnography, 21*(3), 267–306.

Pitts, V. (2003). *In the flesh: The cultural politics of body modification.* New York: Palgrave Macmillan.

Rich, E., & Evans, J. (2013). Now I am nobody, see me for who I am: The paradox of performativity. *Gender and Education, 21*(1), 1–16.

Saba, V. K., & McCormick, K. A. (2001). *Essentials of computers for nurses: Informatics for the new millennium.* New York: McGraw-Hill.

Sassatelli, R. (2010). *Fitness culture: Gyms and the commercialisation of discipline and fun.* Basingstoke: Palgrave Macmillan.

Skarberg, K., & Engström, I. (2007). Troubled social background of male anabolic-androgenic steroid abusers in treatment. *Substance Abuse Treatment, Prevention, and Policy, 2*(20), https://doi.org/10.1186/1747-597x-2-20.

Smith, A. C. T., & Stewart, B. (2012). Body perceptions and health behaviors in an online bodybuilding community. *Qualitative Health Research, 22*(7), 971–985.

Sparkes, A., Batey, J., & Owen, G. (2012). The shame-pride-shame of the muscled self in bodybuilding. In A. Locks & N. Richardson (Eds.), *Critical readings in bodybuilding*. New York: Routledge.

Sykes, G., & Matza, D. (1957). Techniques of neutralization: A theory of delinquency. *American Sociological Review, 22*(6), 664–670.

Thualagant, N. (2012). The conceptualization of fitness doping and its limitations. *Sport in Society: Cultures, Commerce, Media, Politics, 15*(3), 409–419.

Turkle, S. (1995). *Life on screen: Identity in the age of the internet*. London: Weidenfeld and Nicolson.

Wenger, E. (1998). *Communities of practice*. Cambridge and New York: Cambridge University Press.

Part III

Doped Bodies and Gender

7

Re-conceptualizing Doping
and Masculinity

Introduction

In various sporting venues, the construction of masculinity has followed
the imagery of athleticism like a cultural ally for centuries (Guttmann,
1978; Kimmel, 1996; Messner, 1992; Mosse, 1996). By mimicking the
physically demanding practices performed by older men and idols, young
men have been said to internalize normative masculine values through
sport. In addition, devoting time to strengthening the body, building muscles, and projecting an attitude of domination has historically been related
to violence, warfare, and the building of nations, thus implying an interest
in cultivating what Mosse (1996) describes as 'the masculine stereotype.'
The cultural history of contemporary gym and fitness culture is no exception to this kind of cultural narrative (Budd, 1997; Denham, 2008). Klein
(1993), for example, who conducted one of the first bodybuilding studies
in the early 1990s, describes bodybuilding as a predominantly masculine
preoccupation. He also describes homophobia, hyper-masculinity, and the
use of performance- and image-enhancing drugs (PIEDs) as institution-
alized phenomena in this physical culture (see also Locks & Richardson,
2012; McGrath & Chananie-Hill, 2009).

© The Author(s) 2020
J. Andreasson and T. Johansson, *Fitness Doping*,
https://doi.org/10.1007/978-3-030-22105-8_7

The relationship between PIED use and gender is complex. The usual position, in the literature, has been that the main trigger for using PIEDs is men's desire to gain muscle mass and construct a masculine identity (Andreasson & Johansson, 2014; McCreary & Sasse, 2000; Parkinson & Evans, 2006; Sas-Nowosielski, 2006). Looking at previous research on gender and doping, one can see that PIED use has also been understood as an outcome of trying to establish a competitive edge within a sport, as risk-taking, as an integral feature of hegemonic masculinity, and, thus, as an expression of some kind of societal hyper-conformity in relation to constructing masculinity (Andreasson, 2013; Monaghan, 2012; Thualagant, 2012). At the same time, however, PIED use has also been analyzed in terms of deviance and marginalization. It has been connected to mixed abuse, crime, violence, and the margins of society (DuRant, Escobedo, & Heath, 1995; Lentillon-Kaestner & Ohl, 2011).

Using both interview material and online communications, in this chapter we analyze the self-portrayals and gender constructions of male fitness dopers. The aim is to present a dissection and analysis of how fitness doping can be understood in relation to the notion and doing of masculinity. An additional underlying aim is to challenge the notion of masculinity that has traditionally been attached to how fitness doping is understood. Narratives from female users are obviously also of great importance if we wish to challenge popular notions of gender and fitness doping, and this line of inquiry will be developed in Chapter 9.

The chapter is structured as follows. Initially, we present some key theoretical concepts used in the analysis. Next, we present the results, beginning with a section containing some narratives of fitness dopers who can be understood as rather traditional in relation to gender norms and politics. This section thus reveals a historical continuity in the presentation and construction of a muscular masculinity, showing how 'the masculine stereotype' (Mosse, 1996) is reproduced in contemporary fitness culture and through drug use practices. This is followed by two sections in which we use our interview material to investigate different gender configurations. The next section contains online excerpts, and we discuss how the doped hyper-masculine body is negotiated in relation to other masculine positions, for example, that of the male breadwinner and fatherhood. Finally, in the concluding section, we provide a brief and more theoretical summary of the chapter's main contribution to the discussion on doping and masculinity.

Masculinities and the Gender Politics of Fitness Doping

If we are to understand fitness doping in relation to gender, we must dissect the phenomenon in relation to hegemonic masculinity (Connell, 1987, 1995). The concept of hegemonic masculinity was introduced by Connell to describe the hierarchical relations between different masculinities, meaning that there are different ways of enacting manhood and learning how to become a man and that some ways of 'doing' masculinity are dominant while others are marginalized or subordinated. In 1995, Connell defined hegemonic masculinity as a 'configuration of gender practice that embodies the currently accepted answer to the problem of legitimacy of patriarchy' (p. 77; see also Connell & Messerschmidt, 2005). Hence, this concept indicates possible changes in and transformations of gender. Different cultures and periods in history have constructed gender differently, and there is no static pattern of masculinity that can be found everywhere (Connell, 1987).

Hegemony is tightly connected to patriarchy; it is understood as a strategy used to legitimize a particular gender order, as well as a specific constellation of cultural ideals, institutional powers, and politics (Andreasson & Johansson, 2013). The hegemonic position is always contestable, however, and should be viewed as a dynamic concept that suggests possible transformations of gender relations and power structures. Equally important, however, is that we always carefully consider how power hierarchies and power relations are constituted and defined in different contexts and cultures. In contemporary Western societies, not least in a Swedish context, hegemonic masculinity means, for example, being involved, communicative, gender equal, and well-trained, but not too huge or too muscular. As we can see, there is a dynamic interplay between the dominant ideals of masculinity found in society at large and the more specific and subcultural ideals nurtured in certain sociocultural contexts. Bodybuilding culture and fitness doping masculinities may, for example, foster a marginal masculinity involving anti-social activities. Another way of looking at this could be to use the concept of hyper-masculinity, which can be described as a strong exaggeration of certain stereotypical qualities with male connotations, such the emphasis on muscular strength, aggression, sexual virility, and the subordination of women (DeReef, 2006; Mosher & Sirkin, 1984). At the same time, within the subculture, these identities can in fact be combined with a desire to fit into the dominant masculinity (McDowell, Rootham, & Hardgrove, 2014). Furthermore, as suggested by Dahl-Michelsen and Nyheim Solbrække (2014), marginalized masculinities are not only those that do not meet the hegemonic standards, but also those who do not operate in accordance with or make sense of their identities through hegemonic gender norms (see also Anderson, 2009; Cheng, 1999).

In *Inclusive Masculinities*, Anderson (2009) develops a different and rather challenging view of hegemonic masculinity. Anderson suggests that through different social and structural processes—for example, the decline of homophobia—there has been a widening of the range of masculine identities that can be performed and embodied. Although Anderson is aware that many contexts still define masculinity in opposition to femininity and homosexuality, he is quite hopeful when describing a scenario in which masculinity has gradually become more inclusive and accepting. Consequently, inclusive masculinity theory describes the emergence of an archetype of masculinity that undermines the principles of orthodox (read: hegemonic) masculine values, yet one that is also esteemed among male peers (Anderson, 2009; Christensen & Jensen, 2014). Studying gym and fitness culture, however, it is quite obvious that hegemonic masculinity, and the power hierarchies and relations deriving from this structural condition, plays a central role in constituting the identities, relations and subjectivities in this culture. Although we find the theory of inclusive masculinity inspiring, and hopeful, we use these ideas in close connection with feminist theories and different ideas concerning how gender is structured and shaped in contemporary fitness culture.

Analytically, we focus on the dynamic and complex interplay between hyper-masculinity and marginalization, on the one hand, and hegemonic masculinity, on the other. We analyze how the drug use practice is understood and negotiated in relation to different notions of masculinity and how idealized masculinities, when re-contextualized, are seen as marginal or potentially inclusive, and vice versa.

Becoming a Man and the Risk of Losing It All

One significant reason mentioned repeatedly regarding the participants' first involvement in muscle-building practices at the gym is the desire to become stronger, competitive, and to stand out in some way. What we have are the narratives of young men (novices) who to some extent feel physically marginal in relation to the cultural hegemonic ideal and who are seeking ways to become part of it. They are seeking a key to transition from the marginal to the hegemonic body ideal, although through illegal means. Joseph is a good representative of this approach. He started pumping iron at the age of 17 because he found it increasingly difficult to compete and perform physically among his peers. He felt insignificant, like a low achiever in team sports, but in the gym setting, this feeling changed. At the gym, he only had to compete against his own previous results. Joseph explains:

> Well I guess there were some mean kids in my class who went on about me being a bit scrawny, or not very good, but I've never felt like I was totally bullied. (…) I think, what got me started was really, well more an inner ambition or feeling. I thought, I train hard dammit, but I'm never gonna be very good or successful in football, handball, or tennis, or whatever. But here, with the weights, I felt that this is a thing that I could do. I could be the master of my own destiny, so to speak. Back then you didn't know if you had a talent for it, but you kept on training. (Joseph)

Joseph's narrative clearly expresses how a young boy, in his quest to perform and 'hold his ground' in relation to his peers, tries out different paths in life. Thus, Joseph puts forward an ethos that builds on physical strength, masculinity, and the importance of homosocial relations (Kimmel, 1996; Robertson, 2007). This type of ethos is further developed in the following narrative, where PIED use is part of the equation and is perceived almost as a necessary means of upholding a certain way of life and self-understanding.

> Without doping I feel more worn out, torn, and ill. With doping, I feel refreshed and rested. Anyway, there are always gonna be people who think they got it all figured out, right? They usually say things like, 'yeah but it's dangerous' and 'you'll be tempted to use it all the time.' And maybe there are these weak individuals who can't complete a course of treatment and don't know their limits and when to stay clean. But me, when I do treatment courses, I always follow a pattern and a structure. I can always take a break, when I've been on for a certain number of weeks and see that I've had enough for now. If I go over this limit, it is risky, and I might destroy myself. (Robert)

The key concepts in Robert's story are rationality and dominance. His desire to become stronger and develop a muscular body 'that blows everyone away and shocks 'em' made him carefully consider what would be needed to achieve his goals. He entered into the world of steroids and acquired the necessary knowledge to manage and optimize the different courses of treatment in a 'safe' and controlled manner. He distances himself from other users and the non-initiated, presenting himself as rational and in control. Consequently, he is constructing something of a paradigmatic masculine narrative of a successful male career and rationality (Tasker, 1993). He presents a story (a paradigmatic narrative) about a rationalized lifestyle through which he has managed to gradually transform his body from that of a skinny young boy into that of a masculine, competitive, and grown-up man (Hammarén & Johansson, 2014; Messner, 1992; Pronger, 1990).

This can be contrasted with, for example, the experiences of another informant called William. Just like Robert, William started using PIEDs to measure up in comparison with other young men. He started using PIEDs in his twenties when he decided to compete in bodybuilding. At that time, he was quite thin, and he came to realize that he had to engage in drug use practices if he was to assert himself in relation to other bodybuilders on a bodybuilding stage. William's story is somewhat different with regard to the consequences of his drug use practices. For instance, at one point one of the authors (Jesper) sat down with William in the locker room after a joint training session/observation. William was on his way to the showers, when he suddenly stopped in front of Jesper and asked: 'hey, have you seen these.' He pointed at two small scars on each side of his chest, adjacent to his nipples. 'They come from an operation for bitch tits, you know' (gynecomastia). After showering, William brought up the topic again, explaining that at first, he thought the drugs were necessary if he wanted to get any 'real results.' He had never thought much about the possible side effects and risk of this practice. And certainly, he never wanted to develop what he described as 'women's breasts.' Consequently, the initial motives for his drug use resulted in feelings of shame, low self-esteem, and being less of a man—quite the opposite of what he had hoped to achieve (Klein, 1993; Sparkes, Batey, & Owen, 2012). Naturally, the concept of 'bitch tits' and the discussion William pursued could also be situated within a misogynistic discourse and a cultural landscape of oppressive, orthodox masculinity (Anderson, 2009; Saltman, 1998).

It is not surprising that a lifestyle in which the individual customizes his diet, training, and drug regimen and spends countless hours working toward the perfect body also has a great influence on other aspects of social life, in addition to possible drug side effects. Below, Lukas provides an honest description of how problematic it can be to be engaged in fitness doping while in a committed relationship.

> I have this painful memory: my girlfriend is crying and hammering on my chest saying 'I want my old Lukas back.' She saw how I had changed. I was not violent toward her, but she couldn't really reach me, or affect me. So, it has probably been difficult for her. /…/ I went behind her back there, so she took it as a huge betrayal. I can understand that. (Lukas)

Turning his focus to training and building up a solid body, Lukas allowed his girlfriend to become less important. She had seen him grow and had been worried for some time about him starting to use PIEDs to accelerate his physical transformation. Lukas was aware that his girlfriend was worried and tried to conceal his involvement. When she found out, she felt horribly betrayed. This narrative also fits rather neatly into the existing literature on some of the carefully investigated negative effects of steroids and drug use, suggesting that PIED use may cause relationship problems and potentially violent behavior (Bach, 2005; Denham, 2008; DuRant et al., 1995). Although Lukas claims that his experiences with doping never made him violent, he obviously recognizes that the practice changed him and not only in desirable bodily directions (Monaghan, 2001).

Some of the users reported actually having lost control and suggested that their use of PIEDs had made them aggressive. Adrian, for example, explains what happened when he found out that his girlfriend was unfaithful. The interview was conducted just after he got out of jail for the actions described below.

> And then she cheats on me, with my buddy, I mean I was with her for several years. And really, I did anything for her. But then everything just turned black and kind of exploded in my head. So I really beat my friend up bad, and even her, unfortunately. (Adrian)

Now, looking at the situation at a distance, Adrian can see that his girlfriend's unfaithfulness was partly related to him having become something of an unpleasant, controlling person. There is some degree of reflexivity in Adrian's narrative, as there are the other narratives presented above. Still, it is apparent that this kind of domineering masculinity, constructed with the help of PIEDs, feels a constant urge to defend and assert itself—sometimes even with fists, as described above—and to rationalize its own behavior. Consequently, these ways of performing masculinity do not seem to bring about much of a change in the gender politics associated with fitness doping. The fact that some men are willing to use illegal means to achieve the right masculine bodily appearance has been shown in several studies on the prevalence of doping (Andreasson & Johansson, 2017; Christiansen, 2009, 2018; Thualagant, 2012). Furthermore, inherent in the narratives are also the recurring side effects. Here, the desire to continuously develop and become more of a man is countered by the potential risks of consequences that are in direct opposition to those intended, consequences such as loss of control over one's own actions and body in the context of relationships (cf. Denham, 2008). In this sense, there is a delicate balance between the embodiment of normative gender configurations and the inherent threat of 'losing it all' in the pursuit of manhood through drug use practices.

Negotiating Fitness Doping and the Bodybuilding Body

As described and discussed in Chapter 2, gym and fitness culture has gone through a remarkable process of transformation ever since the 1970s (Sassatelli, 2010). The gym has steadily shifted from being perceived as a homosocial and masculine subculture to representing a mass leisure activity (Locks & Richardson, 2012). During this development, typically masculine competitive activities such as bodybuilding have been marginalized (Sassatelli, 2010). In the 1990s, bodybuilding came to be associated with a defensive and compensatory masculinity (Denham, 2008; Klein, 1993). In a Danish study, Mogensen (2011) shows how fitness franchises sometimes use drug tests and anti-doping campaigns with pictures of bodybuilders to maintain their good reputation and eliminate bodybuilders from their clientele. Below, Lars tries to explain how he perceives himself. In his story, it is evident that the identity of a bodybuilder can be highly ambivalent.

> I'm a regular guy who likes to compete in bodybuilding. I think I like doing it and want to continue, but it's not my whole identity, even though I'm immersed in it. But I've always been afraid that people will think that I'm violent or something. 'Cause you know that's what the papers say; people think you're totally whacked out, or look down on others. That you only judge people based on how their body looks. Nah, that's not me. This is something I like to do, and other people can do what they like to do. So I've always been a little afraid that people tend to maybe judge bodybuilders that way. (Lars)

The muscular male body clearly has an ambivalent position in contemporary fitness culture. On the one hand, the lifestyle and dedication to the task that Lars's body represents are highly valued, at least on a cultural and symbolic level. Well-developed and muscular bodies are seen as the outcome of hard-core training and diet and are often displayed in mainstream films as expressing heroic masculinity. On the other hand, the bodybuilding body is often associated with drugs, relationship problems, aggressiveness, and the grotesque, as discussed in the preceding section (see also Locks & Richardson, 2012). Therefore, when positioning himself and his dedication, Lars is clearly careful to project that he is not a freak, an example of what academics have described as 'the postmodern pastiche' (Glasner, 1990). He is a reluctant bodybuilder who wants to present himself in a reflexive manner. Consequently, he is trying to counter populist and mythical descriptions of bodybuilders and PIED users, aiming to widen the stereotypical expectations and conceptions of gender he believes are attached to this practice. In the story below, this negotiating stance is even more explicit.

> Right now, I'm in pretty decent shape. I am 1.9 meters tall and weigh around 135 kilos, so I guess it's pretty obvious that I've been using. But I can sit down and have a conversation, and show that I'm pretty normal anyway, you know. You sit down and eat a hamburger and pizza and stuff like that. You're not extreme or fanatical when it comes to diet. You can have a beer and still talk about alcohol problems in general, you can talk about the situation in Afghanistan, about gender issues, and things like that. (Ted)

Aiming to counter the perceived popular wisdom of other people's (imagined) thoughts about PIED users, Ted tries to present himself not only as a dedicated gym-goer, but also as an intellectual young man. He finds it challenging to control how others perceive him, and when he meets new people, he feels the need to talk about his university studies and show that he is much more than a solid body (cf. Bourdieu, 1984). In some ways, this intellectual, respectable, and reflexive self-portrayal becomes a strategy to counter the stereotypical perception of the bodybuilder as having 'big muscles, no brain,' as Ted puts it (see also Skeggs, 1997).

Another informant, Nicholas, has rather ambitious goals. He has been competing in bodybuilding for a few years, as a heavyweight. He has no problem viewing himself as first and foremost a bodybuilder. His approach to the body is initially centered on constructing a long-term solid and highly muscular body, and this pursuit includes the use of steroids, human growth hormones, and experimentation with insulin. At the same time, his competitive goals and the different seasons of a bodybuilding lifestyle do not always come easy to him. The long-term goals of the training and drug regimen are hard to reconcile with a short-term perspective and an understanding of the self, based on the idea of the body beautiful.

Like now after my last competition, my coach told me I should probably gain some weight, you know, bulk up during the off-season. But I feel that if I'm going to weigh like 125 kilos, I'm going to be really obese. People won't see any difference between me, a bodybuilder, and your average overweight truck driver, and I don't like that. And it's the same before a competition, like on the load-up day. I start at midnight: I get up and eat two burgers with fries and everything. And then I feel like, what the hell am I doing, sitting here wolfing down hamburgers! Because it's a little weird—here I've been eating so healthily for months and suddenly I'm supposed to totally pig out, just to stick to the plan. (Nicholas)

Understanding himself as a healthy young man, Nicholas finds it challenging to justify parts of his diet and body. His focus is on the here and now, on the slender, supple, and muscular body that is primed to be put on display every day of the week. Despite the fact that his lifestyle includes quite advanced courses of PIED treatments in high doses, there is also an aspect of health being negotiated in this narrative that is focused not on the drug regimen, but rather on diet and lifestyle as a whole. In this way, he is writing his own rules for success and formulating a narrative on how to continuously keep fit and look beautiful. Below, these partly 'conflicting,' and traditionally highly gender-binary, perspectives on the body seem to merge, as Andrew describes his perception of training, beauty, and drugs.

It was probably the esthetics and the more symmetrical bodybuilders that inspired me. You know, in beautiful poses and where symmetry and muscle merge into one. It's graceful. /.../ I'm more for the symmetry aspects, the charisma. Like Bob Paris—he was very symmetrical back in the day. But I guess it was also his physical hardness, which is crucial. Plus there was a bit…not just manufactured in the chemical way, but also an incredible discipline. I mean of course it's there, the drugs—otherwise it would never have come so far. You know, like some people think, 'yeah, yeah but you're just on the steroids.' Well, ok, but it's still a lifestyle. (Andrew)

One way of approaching both Andrew's and Nicholas's narratives would be to read them as a normative masculine construction in which the narrator envisions a bodybuilding icon and then based on this icon motivates himself to construct a similar muscular body. These narratives could thus be read as expressions of a man's determination to follow a strictly defined routine to reach the ultimate goal, which is an ideal that coincides with hegemonic masculinity (Connell, 1987, 1995). At the same time, there is also a reflexivity in the excerpts, in which masculinity is constructed in a more sensual and aesthetic manner to represent beauty, charisma, and grace. At stake, here is not only what Andrew wants to create for himself, but also what he finds attractive and impressive.

The fascination with Bob Paris's physicality and the gazing can be read as a manifestation of how the heterosexual gender power order has come to be called into question. It could be understood as an example of what Nixon (1996) describes as a process of cultural transformation in which the bodies of men have come to be sensualized (cf. Rohlinger, 2002). Following this logic, the intense visual monitoring of one's own and other male bodies, the muscles, the shape, and the symmetry, could be understood to some extent as an expression of curiosity about 'the Other' (see also Chapter 5). It could be seen as resulting from increased awareness of the fact that heterosexual men can act in ways once associated with homosexuality, with this now posing less of a threat to their public identity as heterosexuals (Anderson, 2002; 2009). Furthermore, this way of gazing and (symbolically) sensualizing bodies has traditionally been 'reserved for' the bodies of women, and hence, this way of looking at the body could be understood as representing a convergence of male and female physicality (Markula, 2001; Sassatelli, 2010).

Inclusive Masculinities and the Symbolism of Homoerotic Practices

In contemporary gym and fitness culture, the muscular body is idealized and idolized as both an aesthetic and an erotic object. Through the pumping of iron, controlled diets, and sometimes comprehensive drug regimens, the image of the perfect body has been partially revered, as it simultaneously symbolizes hard work and has become a beauty ideal that awakens desires (Sassatelli, 2010). Not surprisingly, this process of cultural transformation has an effect on how people exercise and how they perceive their muscle-building practices. For example, even though the cultural bond between masculinity and muscles has a long history (Kimmel, 1996; Messner, 1992), there are also tendencies toward a convergence of masculinity and femininity. Having a supple, dynamic, and muscular body has become an ideal for both men and women (Bordo, 1990; Johansson, 1996, 1998; Malcolm, 2003; Rohlinger, 2002). This convergence is also evident in some of the narratives presented here. Consider the following narrative, provided by Ian, who has long experience of both competitive bodybuilding and use of PIEDs, when he describes how his perception of gendered bodies manifests itself when he is preparing for a competition.

> You can stand next to the best-looking girl in the world. She could stand there naked even, and you wouldn't see. You don't care either. Like when I'm there it's to be painted, I mean getting your own body tanned or helping someone to put their color on. So it's a different world somehow. (…) If you look at something, it's more like, 'Damn, she's in good shape!' (laughs) It's more like that. (Ian)

Ian defines himself as a heterosexual and is currently engaged to a body fitness competitor. During the bodybuilding and fitness competition from which this narrative derives, however, the object of his desire and the gender of muscles seem to be more fluid and situational in his mind. For example, he describes a situation backstage when he stood in front of a completely naked female fitness competitor engaged in applying bronzers (brown cream) to her inner thighs. His reaction to this 'scenery' was, as he described it, focused on her muscle development. His admiration was not sexual, but rather concentrated on evaluating her level of fitness and symmetry, thus relegating gender (sex) to the background. Naturally, the situation should be understood contextually and is to some extent limited to the bodybuilding scene, given that Ian is engaged to a female fitness competitor. Nevertheless, applying oil and tanning paint close to another person's intimate body parts backstage of the bodybuilding scene, regardless of sex or sexual preferences, could be seen as an act in which the doped, lean, and supple body becomes genderless. It is flesh, beauty, and accomplishment all at once, but not necessarily connected to a specific sex or gender.

The cultural critic Mark Simpson identified what he called the 'metrosexual male' in the mid-1990s (Coad, 2008). What he was trying to describe was a market segment of young urban, predominantly middle-class men preoccupied with appearance, style, and image. When introduced, this phenomenon was thought to indicate a movement toward a new masculinity in crisis, and a closer relationship between homo- and hetero-men (cf. Anderson, 2009). Situated in a gym and fitness context, Ian's narrative, and certainly the following narrative, would fit neatly into such a conception of how the aesthetic and perfectly molded masculine body is understood (cf. Hall, Gough, & Seymour-Smith, 2012).

> But there's this in-betweenness, too, when you talk about it or think about it. It's something not male, but not female either. Or maybe it's gay, actually. Of course, you could see it as being quasi-gay. (Alexander)

Here, Alexander is trying to both understand and problematize his interest in muscular bodies in relation to his gender identity, using the premise that sexual preference is an important expression of masculinity (Fracher & Kimmel, 1995). In his quest for inspiration, 'despite' identifying as heterosexual, he often gazes at other men's bodies, their muscular development, and the shaping and roundness of various body parts. This obviously leads to some reflection and concern. In the following narrative, this way of approaching other men's bodies becomes even more pronounced.

> I think it's a nice feeling. I get so fucking lit. I get turned on when I see people like Joey, when he works out. I really get turned on, well maybe not sexually, but get turned on, on a psychological level. I see him. It is when I see that demon, that's when I'm turned on. (Les)

In Les's narrative, above, the source of his admiration and excitement—the 'turn-on'—is the complete devotion his friends manifest when they work out. But this is also a story about how one man looks at another man in a sensual manner, finding him attractive and beautiful. Although the turn-on is explicitly said to be non-sexual, this way of approaching another man's body could certainly be said to challenge the kind of orthodox masculinity that otherwise typically surrounds gay athleticism and supports hegemonic constructions (Anderson, 2002; Pronger, 1990; Wolf Wendel, Toma, & Morphew, 2001). Both Alexander and Les are in some respect asking themselves whether, given their interest in other men's bodies, they are gay. They do not seem to feel obligated to align their social identity with heterosexuality, nor do they seem to think it is important to avoid being thought of as homosexual men. In this sense, the narratives clearly question the compulsory heterosexuality and homophobia that have served as an ordering principle in many Western cultures, particularly in sports (Anderson, 2009; Klein, 1993; Plummer, 1999). Therefore, on a symbolic level, there is a highly inclusive and also subversive potential in the perspective (read: masculinity) put forward here, in which muscle-building becomes a kind of a motor for changed perspectives in the realm of sexual politics and calling traditional categories of sexual orientation into question (Coad, 2008).

Online Fitness Doping, Career, and Family Life

Whereas the previous sections presenting results have focused on interview and observational material, in this section we return to the online context (introduced in Chapter 6) and take a brief look at how community members on Flashback talk about fitness doping in relation to two central nodes that have historically been closely tied to doing masculinity: making a career/being a breadwinner and being a father. As discussed previously in the chapter, in the interview material presented, it is obvious that the (anticipated) effects of PIEDs are largely connected to the notion of masculinity. This is evident also in the context of online communication. Below, one community member talks about his experiences of PIED use, relating it to thought about masculinity, career, and sexual virility.

> I have experienced really good effects. I've become extremely focused—more of a man. At work, yeah, when I talk, people shut up and show respect. Since my goal in life is to dope myself as much as possible, to achieve as much as possible, I have always seen my job as a parenthetical detail—something you just have to do until you arrive at your real job, the gym. So I've never really invested in pursuing a career. But still, I speak more in front of people.

I have become more sincere and upright. I give and take more (…) not to mention the insane sex drive you get on testo—makes women think you're from Planet Porno. (HeMan)

The above posting vividly captures an understanding of PIEDs that involves an anticipated process of transformation. PIED use is basically connected to adjectives describing the self as becoming more of something, such as more 'focused,' 'muscular,' and 'virile.' Other posters describe how they have developed greater interest in furthering their education, performing at the top of their class in university, and on other arenas. Despite the occasional mention of negative consequences, these qualities are basically described as being desirable. What emerges here is a rational and performance-oriented masculinity. This masculine position is further developed below, where a community member constructs a hypothetical experiment, while simultaneously trying to develop his ideas on the limit-pushing potential of PIEDs.

> Think about this: Wouldn't it be fun to conduct this experiment. Joe works as an officer and his brother works at Lindex [Swedish women's lingerie chain], selling women's underwear. You sneak some estrogen into Joe's coffee and give his brother testo instead. You do this for a couple of months. Talk about different results! What do you think would happen? Yeah, I think I know. In this way we would play out the extremes against each other, to see what really happens, within a particular profession. Testo could be EXTREMELY beneficial.
>
> Ha, ha, yeah, and it would be fun to see the outcome. The total ruin! From officer to army bitch! Ha, ha. I guess the other military boys wouldn't have to pay for porn mags any more. And the brother would probably be reported for sexual harassment at Lindex, found by the surveillance monitors jerking off, while watching the women trying on lingerie in the changing rooms. (TheProfessor)

Although not all of the qualities that come forth are desirable, the outcomes of PIED use are clearly related to a masculine and heterosexual stereotype. Aggressiveness and dominance (or the lack thereof) as well as callous sexual attitudes toward women are constructed as part of a hyper-masculine identity, fueled by testosterone. The imagery of (doped) men at work that emerges in this narrative is thus not constructed in accordance with gender equality and the concept of the communicative, emphatic man. However, while many of the postings seem to rationalize PIED use, constructing it as a masculinity heightener or anchor, there are also narratives in which such use is portrayed as problematic in relation to career choices. This is exemplified in the posting below.

> I actually think it's hard to get anywhere in your career, if we're talking about more qualified jobs. If I were an employer I would probably hesitate before employing a guy who was too big and showed obvious side effects of steroids. Imagine that nice office, and a guy who just wears GASP clothing, because regular shirts don't fit. Hmmm. After all, my experience from different workplaces is that if you look like you're doped, people will say a lot of shitty things behind your back. (TheEmployer)

In the posting above, use of PIEDs is viewed quite pessimistically as regards career advancement. This exemplifies the negotiation between a muscular, dominant hyper-masculinity and what are perceived to be other important aspects of manhood. The doped body, that is, the dominant and intimidating body, is seen here as something that poses a threat to employability and the breadwinner image. Although PIED use is mainly discussed in positive terms on Flashback, it is not always understood as a winning concept. Clearly, how the practice is understood is situated and somehow shifting. This becomes abundantly clear below, where a young single dad, after asking for advice about the risk of losing custody if he were to be caught by the police, tries to explain his perspective on life, drugs, and fatherhood.

> The thing is that I didn't seek out family life. I thought that I would be with my girlfriend for life, that we would get our education and live the life of a child-free couple. Then came the news that she was pregnant, and she wanted to keep it, and my whole world collapsed. I played along for a year. After two years I began to question my life situation on a daily basis. Then I left my family after 2.5 years. Now, I want to start a new life. The plan is to move, get a degree, focus on my training and start a course of steroids. Basically, I want to do what I want, before I start a family (I was 22 when I became a father). Am I selfish leaving my child? Yes, but what

about mothers who give birth to a child against the father's will and think it's going to work? (DaddyNo)

The above posting attracted a great deal of interest. DaddyNo did not, however, get as many comments about custody issues as he had initially hoped. Instead, several members condemned DaddysNo's line of reasoning. To be clear, discussions on Flashback are generally encouraging when it comes to PIED use, but this is obviously not the case when such use is situated like it is in DaddyNo's story. Instead, DaddyNo was strongly advised not to use drugs. Several community members become downright irritated, calling him 'immature' and 'self-centered'—'an idiot with no character.' He is instructed to rethink his priorities in life and to take responsibility for his actions. One community member summarizes the advice contained in the thread by saying: 'Be a man and take care of your child. I know what it means to grow up without a father and I would never expose my own child to that.' Clearly, there are different notions of masculinity being juggled in this discussion of PIEDs and PIED use. The masculine body, the dominant man, the employee, the breadwinner, and the responsible, mature father, in particular, are all integrated into the negotiation of manhood and steroids. The masculinities constructed in the postings are thus understood slightly differently, depending on the situation and how (potential) PIED use is contextualized by the community members.

Conclusions

In this chapter, we have shown how different ideals and notions of masculinity and fitness doping are pitted against each other, and how a marginalized masculinity and identity in the subcultural context are sometimes regarded as constituting a dominant, hegemonic ideal, both in the context of online communication and away from keyboard. Some narratives clearly show how pride in one's physical transformation through PIED use, attainment of an idealized masculinity and symbolically loaded language expressing high expectations can rapidly turn into behavior that is perceived as shameful, when the circumstances are laid out in a problematic way. To this end, the notion of masculinity attached to the understanding of PIED use, as it is expressed, should be understood as an uncertain construction. What makes this even more complex today is the developing fitness trend, which points toward normalization of the hard-core muscle culture cultivated in the fitness and bodybuilding context, leading to shifting attitudes toward drugs, hyper-bodies, and hyper-masculinity in society at large. To a certain extent, we are now seeing how marginalized hyper-masculinity is becoming normalized and incorporated into hegemonic conceptions in mainstream culture; we are simultaneously seeing how a hyper-masculine body is being challenged by other highly valued masculine ideals, such as inclusive and potentially homoerotic masculinity as well as nurturing fatherhood. Thus, what we find here is the possibility to use fitness doping as prism for understanding a variety of positions taken in relation to gender and masculinity.

At least, three distinct and differentiated interpretations or positions seem to emerge through the prism of fitness doping (cf. Braidotti, 1994). The first position, which has been thoroughly described and analyzed in the existing literature, could be described as a *complicit position* in relation to hegemonic masculinity. For example, a common feature of many of the narratives concerning approaches to fitness doping is the underlying idea that the idealized male body can be achieved through continuous effort and with the help of PIEDs. Such a masculinity, constructed in the realm of performance, can clearly be related to a normative masculine stereotype, shaped by traditionalism. Although expressed differently, the overall perspective on masculinity and fitness doping put forward through this position rests heavily on a binary understanding of gendered bodies, doping, and competences, in which the female body is viewed as weak and the male body as strong and competent. Hence, drug use practices are constructed almost solely as a male phenomenon and as heightening masculinity. Consequently, this position situates the bodies of men as inevitably superior to women's bodies within gym culture. In the subcultural context, this position should largely be understood as dominant. However, it also seems as though there is a desire, in some narratives, to expand and exaggerate this position in the direction of certain stereotypical masculine-coded qualities, such as aggression and sexual virility, that constitute a marginalized hyper-masculinity.

The second position that emerges could be described as a negotiating position. On the one hand, this position shows a clear tendency toward complicit masculinities. On the other, it also points in the direction of the transformation of gender configurations and the sexual politics of fitness doping. In many of the narratives that can be situated within this position, the trajectories to drug use seem to originate in quite hegemonic conceptions, such as being motivated by homosocial relationships, etc. At the same time, when we read the narratives, it is clear that such an interpretation is incapable of capturing the entire presentations of the self that are offered and that the narratives have more nuances. These intertwined tendencies are evident when we look at the ways in which some fitness dopers try to 'rewrite' and respond to actual or imagined incidents where their lifestyle choices are called into question. They can be seen in the different ways in which the muscular male body and the body beautiful are explored. They are also manifested in the ways in which use of PIEDs is integrated with the concept of health, intellectualism, involved fatherhood, and more, extending the notion of masculinity and fitness doping in alternative directions.

Finally, we have a more inclusive and potentially subversive position in which fitness doping is renegotiated in relation to the body and heteronormativity (Anderson, 2009). This position emerges when we observe how fitness dopers, regardless of their sexual preferences, can be close to other men and their bodies in a more sensualized, aestheticizing manner. In connection with drug use practices, the focus is so precisely put on the characteristics and shape of the body that, paradoxically, the body itself is detached from sex/gender to some extent. Physicality then becomes more important than sexual orientation, thus enabling men to express emotions and values traditionally associated solely with femininity and/or homosexuality. Consequently, this way of approaching the male body may actually contribute to increased acceptance of, for example, gay identities or other subordinate positions. This approach and position therefore amount to a contestation of hegemonic gender values, in which masculinity and fitness doping have come to be detached from a solidly heterosexual understanding and transformed into inclusiveness and perhaps even homoerotic pleasure, at least on a symbolic level.

Among other things, this chapter reveals the need for future research on fitness doping in relation to gender and sexuality, as well as employability and fatherhood. In addition to continuing our exploration of how fitness doping might be understood and viewed through the prism of masculinity, and the three above-discussed positions, there is also a great need to discuss the experiences and narratives of female PIED users. For this reason, we will look at female users in the next chapter.

References

Anderson, E. (2002). Openly gay athletes: Contesting hegemonic masculinity in a homophobic environment. *Gender & Society, 16* (6), 860–877.

Anderson, E. (2009). *Inclusive masculinities: The changing nature of masculinities.* London: Routledge.

Andreasson, J. (2013). Between performance and beauty: Towards a sociological understanding of trajectories to drug use in a gym and bodybuilding context. *Scandinavian Sport Studies Forum, 4,* 69–90.

Andreasson, J., & Johansson, T. (2013). Female fitness in the blogosphere: Gender, health, and the body. *SAGE Open, 3.* https://doi.org/10.1177/2158244013497728.

Andreasson, J., & Johansson, T. (2014). *The global gym: Gender, health and pedagogies.* Basingstoke, UK: Palgrave Macmillan.

Andreasson, J., & Johansson, T. (2017). Doped manhood: Negotiating fitness doping and masculinity in an online community. In C. Haywood & T. Johansson (Eds.), *Marginalized masculinities: Contexts, continuities and change.* New York and London: Routledge.

Bach, A. R. (2005). *Mænd och muskler: En bog om stryketæning og anabole steroider* [Men and muscles: A book about weight lifting and anabolic steroids]. København, DK: Tiderna skifter.

Bordo, S. (1990). Reading the slender body. In M. Jacobus, F. Keller, & S. Shuttleworth (Eds.), *Body/politics: Women and the discourse of science.* London: Routledge.

Bourdieu, P. (1984). *Distinction: A social critique of the judgement of taste.* London: Routledge.

Braidotti, R. (1994). *Nomadic subjects: Embodiment and sexual difference in contemporary feminist theory.* New York: Columbia University Press.

Budd, M. A. (1997). *The sculpture machine: Physical culture and body politics in the age of empire*. London: Macmillan Press.

Cheng, C. (1999). Marginalized masculinities and hegemonic masculinity: An Introduction. *Journal of Men's Studies, 7*, 295–315.

Christensen, A.-D., & Jensen, S. Q. (2014). Combining hegemonic masculinity and intersectionality. *NORMA: International Journal for Masculinity Studies, 9*(1), 60–75.

Christiansen, A. V. (2009). Doping in fitness and strength training environments: Politics, motives and masculinity. In V. Møller, M. McNamme, & P. Dimeo (Eds.), *Elite sport, doping and public health*. Odense: University Press of Southern Denmark.

Christiansen, A. V. (2018). *Motionsdoping: Styrketræning, identitet og kultur* [Recreational doping: Strenght training, identity and culture]. Aarhus, Denmark: Aarhus Universitetsforlag.

Coad, D. (2008). *The metrosexual: Gender, sexuality, and sport*. New York: Sunny Press.

Connell, R. W. (1987). *Gender & power*. Cambridge: Polity Press.

Connell, R. W. (1995). *Masculinities*. Cambridge: Polity Press.

Connell, R. W., & Messerschmidt, J. W. (2005). Hegemonic masculinity: Rethinking the concept. *Gender & Society, 19*, 829–859.

Dahl-Michelsen, T., & Nyheim Solbrække, K. (2014). When bodies matters: Significance of the body in gender constructions in physiotherapy education. *Gender and Education, 26*, 672–687.

Denham, B. E. (2008). Masculinities in hardcore bodybuilding. *Men and Masculinities, 11*(2), 234–242.

DeReef, J. F. (2006). The relationship between African self-consciousness, cultural misorientation, hypermasculinity, and rap music preference. *Journal of African American Studies, 9*, 45–60.

DuRant, R., Escobedo, L., & Heath, G. (1995). Anabolic-steroid use, strength training, and multiple drug use among adolescents in the United States. *Pediatrics, 96*, 23–29.

Fracher, J., & Kimmel, M. (1995). Hard issues and soft spots: Counselling men about sexuality. In M. Kimmel & M. Messner (Eds.), *Men's lives*. Boston: Allyn and Bacon.

Glasner, B. (1990). Fit for postmodern selfhood. In H. S. Becker & M. M. McCall (Eds.), *Symbolic interaction and cultural studies* (pp. 215–243). Chicago: The University of Chicago Press.

Guttmann, A. (1978). *From ritual to record: The nature of modern sport*. New York: Columbia University Press.

Hall, M., Gough, B., & Seymour-Smith, S. (2012). 'I'm METRO, NOT gay!' A discursive analysis of men's accounts of makeup use on YouTube. *The Journal of Men's Studies, 3*, 209–226.

Hammarén, N., & Johansson, T. (2014). Homosociality: In between power and intimacy. *SAGE Open, 4*. https://doi.org/10.1177/2158244013518057.

Johansson, T. (1996). Gendered spaces: The gym culture and the construction of gender. *Young, 4*(3), 32–47.

Johansson, T. (1998). *Den skulpterade kroppen: Gymkultur, friskvård och estetik* [The sculptured body: Gym culture, wellness and aesthetics]. Stockholm: Carlsson Bokförlag.

Kimmel, M. (1996). *Manhood in America: A cultural history*. New York: The Free Press.

Klein, A. (1993). *Little big men: Bodybuilding, subculture and gender construction.* New York: State University of New York Press.

Lentillon-Kaestner, V., & Ohl, F. (2011). Can we measure accurately the prevalence of doping? *Scandinavian Journal of Medicine & Science in Sport, 21*, 132–142.

Locks, A., & Richardson, N. (2012). *Critical readings in bodybuilding*. New York: Routledge.

Malcolm, N. (2003). Constructing female athleticism: A study of girls recreational softball. *American Behavioral Scientist, 46*(10), 1387–1404.

Markula, P. (2001). Beyond the perfect body: Women's body image distortion in fitness magazine discourse. *Journal of Sport and Social Issues, 25*, 158–179.

McCreary, D., & Sasse, D. (2000). An exploration of the drive for muscularity in adolescent boys and girls. *Journal of American College Health, 48*(6), 297–304.

McDowell, L., Rootham, E., & Hardgrove, A. (2014). Precarious work, protest masculinity and communal regulation: South Asian young men in Luton, UK. *Work, Employment & Society, 28*, 847–864.

McGrath, S., & Chananie-Hill, R. (2009). 'Big Freaky-Looking Women': Normalizing gender transgression through bodybuilding. *Sociology of Sport Journal, 26*, 235–254.

Messner, M. (1992). *Power at play: Sports and the problem of masculinity*. Boston: Beacon Press.

Mogensen, K. (2011). *Body Punk: En afhandling om mandlige kropsbyggere og kroppens betydninger i lyset av antidoping kampagner* [Body punk: A thesis on male bodybuilders and the meanings of the body in the light of anti-doping campaigns]. Roskilde: Roskilde Universitetscenter.

Monaghan, L. F. (2001). *Bodybuilding, drugs and risk: Health, risk and society*. New York: Routledge.

Monaghan, L. F. (2012). Accounting for illicit steroid use: Bodybuilders' justifications. In A. Locks & N. Richardson (Eds.), *Critical readings in bodybuilding*. New York: Routledge.

Mosher, D. L., & Sirkin, M. (1984). Measuring a macho personality constellation. *Journal of Research in Personality, 18*, 150–163.

Mosse, G. (1996). *The image of man: The creation of modern masculinity*. New York and Oxford: Oxford University Press.

Nixon, S. (1996). *Hard looks: Masculinities, spectatorship & contemporary consumption*. London: UCL Press.

Parkinson, A. B., & Evans, N. A. (2006). Anabolic androgenic steroids: A survey of 500 users. *Medicine and Science in Sport and Exercise, 38*(4), 644–651.

Plummer, D. (1999). *One of the boys: Masculinity, homophobia and modern manhood*. New York: Harrington Park Press.

Pronger, B. (1990). *The arena of masculinity: Sports, homosexuality, and the meaning of sex*. New York: St. Martin's.

Robertson, S. (2007). *Understanding men and health: Masculinities, identity and well-being*. Berkshire: Open University Press.

Rohlinger, D. A. (2002). Eroticizing men: Cultural influences on advertising and male objectification. *Sex Roles, 46*(3), 61–74.

Saltman, K. (1998). Men with breasts. *Journal of the Philosophy of Sport, 25*, 48–60.

Sas-Nowosielski, K. (2006). The abuse of anabolic-androgenic steroids by Polish school-aged adolescents. *Biology of Sport, 23*(3), 225–235.

Sassatelli, R. (2010). *Fitness culture: Gyms and the commercialisation of discipline and fun*. London: Palgrave Macmillan.

Skeggs, B. (1997). *Formations of class and gender: Becoming respectable*. London: Sage.

Sparkes, A., Batey, J., & Owen, G. (2012). The shame-pride-shame of the muscled self in bodybuilding. In A. Locks & N. Richardson (Eds.), *Critical readings in bodybuilding*. New York: Routledge.

Tasker, Y. (1993). *Spectacular bodies: Gender, genre and the action cinema*. New York: Routledge.

Thualagant, N. (2012). The conceptualization of fitness doping and its limitations. *Sport in Society: Cultures, Commerce, Media, Politics, 15*(3), 409–419.

Wolf Wendel, L., Toma, D., & Morphew, C. (2001). How much difference is too much difference? Perceptions of gay men and lesbians in intercollegiate athletics. *Journal of College Student Development., 42*(5), 465–479.

8

Female Fitness Doping

Introduction

Scholars' interest in women's use of performance- and image-enhancing drugs (PIEDs) in the context of gym and fitness culture has come to focus mainly on female bodybuilders (McGrath & Chananie-Hill, 2009). Female bodybuilding essentially began in the late 1970s (Fair, 1999). In the 1980s and 1990s, highly muscular and defined female bodies gradually gained recognition, both within bodybuilding and in the public discourse. As these women's bodies steadily grew in mass and vascularity, discussions on PIEDs also emerged. Little by little, women entered the subculture of male bodybuilding, including adopting the drug use practices associated with this culture (Liokaftos, 2018). Gender transgressions rarely go unnoticed, however. Women's muscle-building, particularly through drug use practices, has therefore often been considered a threat to the 'natural' gender order (Richardson, 2008). This applies particularly to women's gender border-crossing into the realm of muscular masculinity (Aoki, 1996; McGrath & Chananie-Hill, 2009). Regarding women's use of prohibited substances and muscle-building practices, scholars have also debated whether they are to be understood as gender transgressions or

© The Author(s) 2020
J. Andreasson and T. Johansson, *Fitness Doping*,
https://doi.org/10.1007/978-3-030-22105-8_8

whether they merely reinforce already existing polarized understandings of gender. As suggested by McGrath and Chananie-Hill (2009), the answer to this complex question is slippery and resists definitive analysis, as do other social issues requiring 'both/and' discourses, rather than 'either/or' binaries. The initial answer to this question has thus been that women's muscle-building practices, particularly those involving fitness doping, act as a subversive and empowering force and reinforce normative gender configurations (Boyle, 2005; Hill Collins, 2000; Roussel, Monaghan, Javerlhiac, & Yondre, 2010).

Continuing this line of discussion, in this chapter we look at Swedish female PIED users' narratives. Using qualitative interview material gathered in the context of gym and fitness culture and data from various postings from the pro-doping online community Flashback, our aim is to describe and analyze how female PIED users understand and negotiate their use of PIEDs. Studies on women's PIED use in the context of gym and fitness culture have focused largely on female bodybuilders. While this study, too, includes narratives from bodybuilders, the sampling also includes narratives from fitness competitors and temporary female users (see Chapter 10 for further information). We are interested in the reactions the participants experience regarding female muscularity, in general, and women's PIED use, in particular. We are also interested in the meanings the women ascribe to fitness doping in relation to their own understanding of gender and the body.

The chapter is structured as follows: In the next section, we describe the general background of the chapter. Next, in the results sections, we present and analyze excerpts from interviews and online postings, addressing the above-described aims. Finally, in the concluding section, we provide a condensed and more theoretical summary of the chapter's main outcomes.

Enter: Female Bodybuilders

In gym and fitness culture, the relationship between gender, strength training, and PIED use has largely been a story about male bodybuilders, their muscles and masculinity (Christiansen, 2018; Denham, 2008; Klein, 1993; Liokaftos, 2018; Monaghan, 2001, 2012). Scholars have also concluded that, in the Western world, use of PIEDs by those who practice strength training is more common among men than among women (Breivik, Hanstad, & Loland, 2009; Christiansen 2018; Sagoe, Andreassen, & Pallesen, 2014). Furthermore, and as described in Chapter 2, *The International Federation of Bodybuilding and Fitness* (IFBB), which is the governing body of the sport of bodybuilding and fitness, has insisted that women should maintain their 'female forms' and femininity (IFBB, 2018). Introducing new disciplines, such as *Women's Bikini-Fitness* and *Women's Wellness Fitness*, and simultaneously limiting competitions in female bodybuilding—strong incentives to influence (limit) the development of women's muscle-building and fitness doping—have thus been put forward by central stakeholders and policymakers within the IFBB. Nevertheless, the female bodybuilders of the 1990s brought new ideals forward (Lindsay, 1996). For instance, the female slimness ideal has shifted toward that of a lean, athletic, fit, and strong female physique and body ideal (Grogan, 2006). This is abundantly clear in the highly promoted notion of 'strong is the new skinny' that is prevalent in popular media and heavily marketed on various *fitspiration webpages* (Boepple, Ata, Rum, & Thompson, 2016; Sassatelli, 2010). According to Van Hout and Hearne (2016), this shift in female muscularity and the female body ideal has also potentially contributed to women adopting specific behaviors that have male connotations in relation to drug supplementation and fitness training (see also Field et al., 2005; Muller, Gorrow, & Schneider, 2009).

Although there are indications of increasing social acceptance in society as a whole, and particularly in fitness culture, as regards women's muscle-building practices, women's engagement in fitness doping has still largely escaped scholarly attention (Evans-Brown & McVeigh, 2009; Van Hout & Hearne, 2016). Research also shows that drug supplementation (PIED use) differs by gender (Andreasson & Johansson, 2014; Klein, 1993). Whereas men have had access to online forums and subcultural settings in which PIED use is discussed (Monaghan, 2012; Smith and Stewart, 2012), women have largely been left out of such supportive and social communities (Griffet, 2000; Thualagant, 2012; Van Hout & Hearne 2016). Bunsell (2013) discusses this in relation to a veil of secrecy and a taboo, through which women have come to underplay their use of PIEDs and been forced to trust others (read: men) to guide them in their fitness doping practices (see also McGrath & Chananie-Hill, 2009). Due to the historical association between muscles and masculinity, women are also more likely to use supplements considered 'less masculine,' such as human growth hormones (HGH), ephedrine and clenbuterol, as opposed to muscle-enhancing supplements such as steroids (Jespersen, 2012). Existing research on female users also indicates that women's motives for engaging in drug use have centered on, among other things, weight loss, muscle enhancement, youthful skin, improved sleep, and injury healing (Van Hout & Hearne, 2016). In a similar vein, Baker, Graham, and Davies (2006) found increases in use of growth hormone for cosmetic reasons among female gym-goers, with particular sourcing routes grounded in Internet retail. Utilizing a netnographic approach, this study touches on the emerging trend of women using growth hormones for anti-aging, lipolysis, and rehabilitation purposes. Of course, these patterns also correspond to the (gendered) side effects associated with the various substances. Although female fitness doping should be considered under researched, the times are changing.

> Use of enhancement drugs among women involved in recreational fitness training and willingness to share opinions and information on the Internet have been observed in recent times, and are perhaps indicative of diffusion of drug enhancement supplements into more mainstream female groups interested to discover the world of image and performance enhancement. (Van Hout & Hearne, 2016, p. 8)

A Silent Revolution

The discussion on how the fitness body is socially constructed and how power relations are inscribed on the body also suggests that the flesh is the starting point of a discussion on how to counteract and eventually change social representations. Feminism has been successful in bringing forward theoretical tools and conceptual frameworks that can be used to present and analyze alternative representations and images of gender and identity. The desire to influence, change and possibly even revolutionize gender relations and society is highly prominent in the writings of many contemporary feminist writers, such as in the American feminist and historian Donna Haraway's science and technology studies, especially her now classical writings from the 1990s on the cyborg. Cyborgs are portrayed as a complex synthesis of organic and synthetic parts. These fictional figures are often used to portray the question of the difference between human and machine as a question concerned with morality, free will, and emotions. The cyborg has become something of the admass society's root metaphor, that is, a metaphor that comprises several key aspects of contemporary society. This metaphor functions as a tight composite picture of the extended and nearly extinguished self. It blurs the boundaries between nature and culture, man/woman and machine, reality and illusion. Given that the metaphor is useful for pointing out a number of boundary transgressions, it also functions well as a guide to the current state of *liquid modernity*.

This subversive tradition is also well represented by the American feminist Judith Butler, who claims that the notions of masculinity and femininity, indeed the heterosexual order, are social and cultural constructions (Butler, 1990, 1993, 2004). Such an assumption constitutes a starting point from which to question the prevailing outlook on gender, sexuality, and identity. In order to theorize about sexuality and gender, Butler uses several examples and case studies of people who have broken with the predominant gender and sexuality order. She claims that these cases show how fragile and unstable the gender order is. Transvestites, female bodybuilders, bisexuals, and other positions viewed as 'deviant' in the public discourse reveal the extent to which gender is a game, an act, and how everything is based on a well-developed dramaturgy. According to Butler, however, it is extremely difficult to change people's conceptions of gender and sexuality. These conceptions are inscribed in the body and deeply rooted in society and the individual psyche. The discovery that gender is not an essential feature, therefore, constitutes merely the first step toward real change. When people dare to violate the gender order, the boundaries suddenly become visible. Sometimes we convince ourselves that we are freer than we actually are. Such an illusion is shattered, however, when we suddenly see how the system both produces and punishes deviants.

Listening to the stories of the women interviewed, and reading the postings on Flashback, we are taking part in a *silent revolution*. Female bodies are molded and shaped in new ways, through muscle-building practices and fitness doping. Through new body techniques and refined training schedules, extreme bodies are created, and the limits of the flesh perforated. In many respects, women who started doing bodybuilding in the late twentieth century paved the way for contemporary women to pursue strength training and other activities aimed at changing the constitution of the body. The negative reactions to female bodybuilders in the 1990s were ruthless. Crossing a boundary is never easy. Looking at the bigger picture, however, we can establish that the majority of individuals who engage in bodybuilding, and have the time to build extreme bodies through drug use practices, are still men. Still, we argue that it is important to try to discern and interpret signs of ongoing sociocultural changes and transformations of the gender balance in society by studying female fitness dopers. Butler (1990, p. 29) states that 'Fantasy is not the opposite of reality; it is what reality forecloses, and, as a result, it defines the limits of reality, constituting it as its constitutive outside. /.../ Fantasy is what allows us to imagine ourselves and others otherwise; it establishes the possible in excess of the real; it points elsewhere, and when it is embodied, it brings the elsewhere home.'

PIED Use, the Law, and the Other Gender

The Swedish Doping Act (1991:1969), which was adopted by the Riksdag and brought into effect in 1992, made it possible to intensify Swedish anti-doping work by criminalizing the use and possession of doping substances and by implementing stricter criminal penalties. Therefore, we can safely say that, in the Swedish context since the 1990s, PIED use has been viewed as a public health issue and societal problem. As touched on in Chapter 7, this problem has primarily been discussed in relation to young men's muscular masculinities, particularly in the public discourse (Andreasson, 2015). Although acceptance of extreme bodies and different ways of 'doing gender' are more common in the public discourse today, women's fitness doping practices have been marginalized not only due to effects of the Swedish Doping Act, but also due to the gendered expectations attached to the practice. This, of course, also influences users' understandings of PIEDs and how they negotiate their lifestyle.

One of the participants, Mathilda, is 33 and works as a housing agent. Her interest in strength training has developed over a long period. Initially, she mostly participated in group fitness activities, but after a couple of years of going to her local gym, her interest in strength training grew. She was fascinated by how her body and its constitution changed, how body fat gradually disappeared and was replaced with muscles. She wanted to create a lean, slim, and muscular physique, but this gradually changed into a desire to compete in bodybuilding. In the following excerpt, she describes how this desire was fulfilled, and her feeling of being constantly scrutinized at the gym, due to her muscular body:

> People think you're stupid, doing bodybuilding. Even at SATS, which is a regular gym, you're doomed. When they see that you lift a little heavier than a regular person might do in a gym, they just stare at you. I used to train at World Class gym before. When we met and had a chat a month ago, that was actually one of the first times I was here that week. Usually I'm only here on weekends, with Chris. However, you know, I got such strange stares at the end of the week, from the regulars who work out here. Also, I try to dress as femininely as possible at my job. I usually wear a dress or a skirt. I think I try to hide myself a bit, to make it less confrontational. So they won't think, 'Oh my God - she looks like a transvestite.' Or, 'Damn she has really been working out and used drugs and all that.'

Mathilda describes feelings of being *otherized* and gazed at, not only when working out at the gym, but also at work. To avoid being treated as an outsider, she tries to adjust the way she presents herself to accord with general perceptions of how women should dress and act. The 'uncanny Other' is present here as a 'steroid-filled transvestite.' This feeling of being misunderstood and gazed at is quite common among the women interviewed. Whereas the fitness-doping men and their muscles are understood as being somewhat in sync with idealized notions of muscular masculinities, there are no obvious cultural alliances between femininity and muscles. This kind of narrative also resonates well with the research on female athletes, showing how they are socially excluded or framed within polarized gender configurations and discourses of emphasized femininities (Bolin & Granskog, 2003; Malcolm, 2000).

Although the women interviewed are highly aware that their bodies and drug use practices can be seen as extreme, in relation to not only flouting Swedish law, but also gender transgression, they also yearn for recognition and to be treated as normal/ordinary. Another participant explains:

> Well, there are people who are impressed and think it's fun, but that is a small crowd. One also gets many negative reactions, draining your energy levels. I just want people to realize that I'm only a human, as if I could explain: 'Yeah, I can see it in your eyes, what you think of me.' I mean, it's not as if I'm this unbelievable robot, just because I'm really pumped up and defined in my workout. I'm just struggling so hard. And actually, what you want is just to have some rewards, instead of all these negative reactions. It's a pity because I don't think people really understand the amount of hard work that goes into this body. They just see the freak working out in the gym. When you're working out, your muscles are veined and strained. It looks extreme. (Liz)

The experience of being treated differently and seen as somehow deviant is present in several narratives. Narratives of extreme bodies are also intertwined with narratives of drug use. In a way, as implied above, use of PIEDs is thought to colonize other people's opinions about femininity and muscles, concealing the tremendous effort and time invested in training and diet (Monaghan, 2001). Another participant, Catherine, has been professionally involved in bodybuilding for many years. She also talks about the regular checks made as a form of harassment.

> I don't care that much, but the thing is that they take away your driving license. Some of my friends were harassed one morning. They had this 'Operation Liquid' at six o'clock in the morning. One of my friends was asleep in Gothenburg when they attacked. They were looking for her boyfriend. She was asleep, and he was not even there, but they kicked in the door - six cops with their weapons drawn. She was about to wet herself! I just say, if you're active in an organization and competing, they will have drug tests, and that's fine. You will not get a fine if you test positive at a competition, but if they pass on that information, you'll lose your driver's license. Why involve the police? (Catherine)

The above narrative obviously needs to be understood in relation to the national context and the strong preventative measures that have been implemented to stop both trafficking of PIEDs and use of these drugs in Sweden. In this context, Catherine, like others, expresses feelings of humiliation and being otherized in daily life. However, this is connected not only to the fact that engaging in drug use practices means breaking (and questioning) the law, but also to their understanding of gender and femininity. When talking about it, they envision the female PIED user as a 'gender bender' and a transgressive gestalt. At the same time, they also express a desire to fit in, to be seen/accepted as ordinary (read normal) and to be part of society. What the women describe is how their lifestyle choices are received by others, and they also touch on their experiences of being seen as outsiders. Through their practices, they are apparently breaking boundaries and challenging gender norms and performative codes in society, as well as the law. In one sense, this can be seen as a semi-rebellious act that empowers female muscularity as a cultural ideal (Grogan, Evans, Wright, & Hunter, 2004; McGrath & Chananie-Hill, 2009). At the same time, this is more an effect of their presence in mainstream gym and fitness culture and society, as these women do not seem to aspire to transgressing gender or confronting stereotypical gender ideals. Instead, their wish is to be respected/accepted while trying to maintain a certain lifestyle, including using PIEDs and developing bulky muscles on a female body.

Accepting the Rules of the Game

Since the 1990s, women have had difficulty being accepted in the realm of competitive and male-dominated bodybuilding. While female bodybuilding is still largely marginalized, new forms of female body ideals have evolved that are more open to (moderate) muscular femininities. This is exemplified in the narrative of Erika, below. She is 20 years old and has gradually become seriously involved in strength training and *Bodyfitness*. Although this competitive discipline includes assessments of women's self-presentation, grace, hair, makeup, and personal confidence, all of which have connotations to femininity, it also has many similarities to traditional bodybuilding, in which the overall athletic appearance of the physique is evaluated in terms of muscle tone/development, body fat, and symmetry (IFBB, 2018). Additionally, questions that concern the shaping of a bodyfitness body are evidently also questions that concern PIED use. Erika describes how her image of the fitness culture gradually changed, especially concerning the use of drugs.

> Therefore, because I'm so fresh, I've been naive from the start. I have to admit that. Now I have a completely different view, compared to what I had a year ago. I know how it works, and it's a bit more like if you're in the game, then you also have to play and endure the game. So, if you look at sports or if we talk about drugs and sport, then I seriously thought that people who competed and won were clean. I thought you could do that. However, I've been told that it is just rumors. You get a different view when talking to people now. There is a completely different attitude toward drugs among people, but now I also know more about how it works. (Erika)

Although Erika is not involved in bodybuilding, she is participating in the same cultural space as male and female bodybuilders and is thus drawn into the discussion on PIEDs. When she talks about 'people,' it is her training friends and fellow competitors she has in mind. Aiming to become a fitness competitor, she gradually realizes what she needs to be prepared to do in order to reach this goal. She also admits that her attitude toward PIEDs has recently changed; she has become more accepting. Another participant continues:

> I believe there are PIEDs that work better, causing no direct harm, helping the individual to progress. I also understand that you need to use extra facilitators to reach higher levels. When you reach a certain level, or a plateau, where your training and results stagnate, you just feel restless. You want to reach higher levels more rapidly. Well, it's simpler then, and you still love it. (Ruth)

What Ruth exemplifies is a habituation process through which growing ambition and more intense training schedules gradually come to include PIED use. The training repertoire is in a way intact, but new 'formulas' are added. Another woman, Mathilda, is of the same opinion. She is trying to soften the image of the 'PIED-using lazy bodybuilder.' Although not trying to downplay the role of PIEDs in the culture and bodily projects, she wants to put forward a more complex image of the/her lifestyle. The ethos she presents is characterized primarily by discipline, diet, asceticism, and a lifestyle in which people are ready to sacrifice everything in order to reach their goals.

> Well, it's just a myth that muscles pop up by themselves and that you are ready in one month's time, just because you use a lot of different drugs. People are actually sacrificing their social life. If you're in a relationship, for example, you have to sacrifice a lot of the usual aspects of everyday life, you know. Therefore, you put a lot of energy into it, both mentally and physically. I think it's important to get the whole picture - that there is a lot of work behind the progress made: you're not just sitting there getting stronger and stronger by stuffing yourself with drugs. (Mathilda)

What we notice here is a gradual acceptance of PIEDs, and a growing inclination to justify and rationalize its use. Different motivations are expressed, and physiological and psychological boundaries are challenged. This can also be interpreted as an effect of women increasingly becoming part of the inner circle of the fitness community, in which PIED use is more broadly tolerated, if not entirely accepted. No longer at the margins of bodybuilding and fitness culture, the women interviewed have a partly strained, partly relaxed view of PIEDs. They share a widespread acceptance of using PIEDs to reach higher performance levels and win competitions. They also defend the subcultural ethos of bodybuilding. At the same time, fitness doping is seen as just one part of a larger picture in which discipline, diets, and hard training are the most important parts. Furthermore, in terms of gender and femininity, the use and effects of the drugs are often understood as complicated and complex.

Approaching PIEDs in the Context of Online Communication

Based on the experiences described in the narratives above, in this section approach how female PIED users talk about their drug use practices in the context of online communication. In order to analyze the women's approaches, we will use a number of excerpts from discussions on the Swedish online community Flashback. One advantage of this form of data collection is that it is often possible to view members' postings over several years. Thus, one can see how they initially approach PIEDs, and perhaps later initiate the practice.

PeptideJudy has been a member of Flashback since 2014. In one of her initial postings connected with the theme of *Training*, she asks for advice on how to gain muscle mass and about others' experiences of different personal trainers. At this point, she has no particular interest in PIED use (not on Flashback at least). About a year later, however, we can read that she has still not found a personal trainer and has therefore decided to 'try the chemical way' to reach her goals. She initiates a new discussion, this time on the theme of *Doping*:

> I'm going to start a new course of peptides on Monday. This is my plan, please comment☺. I will go for HGH, 176-191, comes from Gen-Shi Labs. I've got some other stuff too, but I'm not gonna do that now. My goal is to lose weight and simultaneously build/keep some muscles. /.../ I went through a period in my life (not gonna tell you what) that made me gain weight. I've tried almost everything to lose weight. I'm an all-or-nothing girl, so starting Monday I'm gonna give it everything I've got. (PeptideJudy)

A few days after the above excerpt was posted, we read how PeptideJudy informs her readers that she has now 'taken HGH every morning for three days' and although she has felt a little light-headed, she is mainly positive about her partly new routine. Moving on, after another three months, PeptideJudy evaluates her development and concludes that her course of human growth hormones (HGH) helped her tighten her body, but due to financial constraints she has decided to try to focus exclusively on training and diet. What this narrative/case shows is that the process of engaging in PIED use cannot always be neatly attached to prolonged strategies to reach competitive bodily levels in bodybuilding or body fitness. Rather, for PeptideJudy, engagement in PIED use seems to have been triggered when other means (e.g., using a personal trainer) failed. Further, at some point, after achieving a certain level of success, she could not find sufficiently strong financial arguments for continued use. What is exemplified here, then, is a temporary and recreational meaning-making strategy and doping trajectory (Christiansen, 2018).

Below, another female community member, called *the Winstrol-lady*, explains her rationale for engaging in a course of steroids (Winstrol). She explains that she used to have a rather unhealthy lifestyle, including use of both alcohol and pot, but she has now decided she wants to turn her life around. After one week on steroids, she explains the following regarding her use, the meanings attached to it and how it affects her:

> Is it possible to feel results already? I woke up this morning and felt like I had to rape the first man I met. Luckily, there was one lying right next to me /… / I felt happy and comfortable in my body the whole day. I don't know if it's a placebo effect, or the lovely weather, being spring and all that. Anyhow, I feel like a new human being and kind of have restless legs. However, there are no obvious improvements in my training. Maybe I should add, though, that I'm starting to feel that my body is firmer, especially my ass and thighs. Overall, I'm happy, horny and hungry, on exercise and good food. (the Winstrol-lady)

As exemplified above, one tendency regarding use is that the women's reports are quite optimistic. Their narratives express happiness, and encouraging testimonies regarding the effects of the drugs. It is also clear that the female users are becoming more a part of, and more used to the rationales of, the fitness doping community on Flashback. Although it still seems to be the case that men support and to a certain degree teach women about how to approach and use various drugs, the women are also gradually becoming more independent in combining training schedules and use of PIEDs. *BodyCheat*, for example, describes how her partner led the way to fitness doping, and how she is somewhat of a novice at the gym. At the same time, she is very clear about what she wants to accomplish:

> Of course, my partner helps me there, and his advice is welcome, naturally. My partner has developed a schedule for my diet. I know what I want, at least. I do not want the body of a 12-year-old. But, sure, weight training is new to me. But I will learn, you will see. I am 37 years old. I'm not a

teenager who wants to be cool, with lots of muscles. I want a body I can enjoy. In addition, if I need to cheat to get there, I'll do it. (BodyCheat)

In contrast to parts of the interview material presented earlier, we also find narratives from women who use PIEDs occasionally. The postings on Flashback show that these women are prepared to use PIEDs to achieve a more well-defined and stronger body, but they are not talking about becoming female bodybuilders or, as another community member expressed it, a 'stereotypical fitness nerd.' Instead, these women mainly want to improve their bodies to a certain extent, to reach a certain level. For some women, a single course proves sufficient. For others, of course, the levels are constantly shifting. Below, one woman who initially wanted to lose weight, but after her first course also wanted to compete, talks about the role of fitness doping when one aims to be a *Bikini-Fitness* competitor:

> The results came relatively fast. The star of this development is mainly Anavar. I have become a lot harder during these past few weeks—my upper body is almost finished. My lower body takes a bit longer because that's where most of my fat is, but the fronts of my thighs and my butt are really shaping up. The downside of having introduced clenbuterol a little late is that I collected some fluids on Anavar, especially after I raised it from 20 to 40 per day. So it got a little confused for a while, as the scale suddenly showed a couple of extra hectograms. Now, when the clenbuterol has kicked in, I've begun to release some fluid. I've added ephedrine to the course and combine these three. But, at the same time, I've been on and off the clenbuterol to avoid damaging my heart (3 days on, 3 days off). (TheDoctor)

Exemplified here are not only rigorous experiences of combining different kinds of substances, but also—in the subsequent postings in this thread—detailed advice on how other women can learn from the courses described. Flashback thus enables presumptive female users to find advice on how they can approach and use PIEDs. There is serious expertise and advice to be found on Flashback, although the question of the soundness of this advice is not always considered. Nevertheless, whereas women in the 1980s and 1990s had difficulty finding advice in the form of different course reports related to their needs, today there is a vast amount of information. This also points to the increased integration of women into the communities, as well as the gradually more advanced use of PIEDs to promote 'better bodies' and to reach higher levels of female achievement. This development of female expertise and advice is exemplified in the excerpt below, in which one community member initiates a thread encouraging other women to ask her advice regarding PIED use and 'women's issues':

> Do you have any 'sensitive' questions about the use of doping and being a woman? Feel free to send me questions. I have a medical background and I plan my own courses, so I should be able to answer most things, if you want to know. I was thinking about initiating a new course on Monday, as it seems now. It will be a little different from last time, 24 weeks total. (WomensIssuesMD)

While the excerpt above shows a gradual shift toward more gender-neutral communities in which men and women can discuss their similar as well as different experiences of PIED use and of the effects of use, this is still a world dominated by men. To this end, and although there is a large number of threads concerning drug using practices on Flashback, it is most often taken for granted that the advice and course reports are written for and by men. Many of the female users identified also mention the difficulty of finding course reports from other women. However, this subfield of drug use practices is gradually changing.

Conclusions

Given that a shame threshold for women using PIED still exists, gaining access to personal narratives proved difficult. For this chapter, combining empirical material from different sources—interviews and an Internet forum—was seen as a possible solution to studying practices that have largely been understudied in the existing literature. Through biographical narratives and online postings, we have focused on female PIED users and how they understand and negotiate their use of PIEDs in relation to female muscularity and gender. The analysis reveals that, in their daily lives, the female users' initiation of drug use is largely connected to the cultural framing of gym and fitness. This use is connected particularly to the women's developing thoughts about muscular femininities and to their, possibly unintended, challenging of the normative structures of hegemonic masculinities.

The face of gym and fitness has changed in recent decades, and it is possible to talk about a globalized fitness revolution. One fascinating part of this cultural transformation concerns the strained but also independent relationship that has developed between bodybuilding and fitness. Whereas bodybuilding is still considered suspect and related to drugs, fitness has been associated with health and sound lifestyles. This chapter, however, indicates that the lines between bodybuilding (with male connotations) and physical fitness/wellness have become less clear. Although bodybuilding is largely marginalized in contemporary fitness culture, competitive bodies, associated with drug use practices, are cherished at the same time, in terms of their lifestyle-forming practices.

The gender of muscularity is gradually changing, and idealized notions of female muscularity are becoming more acceptable. In this sense, strong is truly becoming the new skinny. Although not uncontested, traditional standards of femininity are being challenged, and the narratives presented in this chapter exemplify the slow but growing acceptance of muscular female bodies constituted within the 'normal' range of femininity (McGrath & Chananie-Hill, 2009). This would also seem to pave the way for more liberal and accepting attitudes toward use of PIEDs among women. In this respect, our female PIED users are in a unique position. On the one hand, their narratives on muscular femininities exemplify freedom of gender expression and transgression. On the other, the women are also finding that their PIED use practices are questioned not only in relation to breaking the law, but also in relation to a fairly robust gender order. In this respect, our study corresponds to and can thus be situated in relation to the research on female bodybuilders conducted mainly in the 1990s and early 2000s, although the doping demography represented here is somewhat broader.

Although this chapter has presented a small and limited investigation, we suggest that the results attest to the importance of acquiring further knowledge on the gendered structure of PIED use in contemporary society. Although PIED use in the context of gym and fitness culture remains principally a masculine domain, our results point to a development in which women are increasingly being invited to join and integrated into a community of PIED users. For example, they are not dependent on men to obtain information and drug reports, and there is an increasing amount of knowledge on the Internet that is not only aimed at, but has also been developed by and for women. Future research would benefit from a more in-depth investigation into the effects this development has on the gendered dimensions of fitness doping demographics, in general, and female fitness doping trajectories, in particular.

References

Andreasson, J. (2015). Reconceptualising the gender of fitness doping: Reconceptualising the gender of fitness doping—Performing and negotiating masculinity through drug-use practices. *Social Sciences, 4,* 546–562.

Andreasson, J., & Johansson, T. (2014). *The global gym: Gender, health and pedagogies.* Basingstoke, UK: Palgrave Macmillan.

Aoki, D. (1996). Sex and muscle: The female bodybuilder meets Lacan. *Body & Society, 4,* 59–74.

Baker, J. S., Graham, M. R., & Davies, B. (2006). Steroid and prescription medicine abuse in the health and fitness community: A regional study. *European Journal of Internal Medicine, 17*(7), 479–484.

Boepple, L., Ata, R. N., Rum, R., & Thompson, K. (2016). Strong is the new skinny: A content analysis of fitspiration websites. *Body Image, 17,* 132–135.

Bolin, A., & Granskog, J. (2003). *Athletic intruders: Ethnographic research on women, culture, and exercise.* New York, NY: State University of New York.

Boyle, L. (2005). Flexing the tensions of female muscularity: How female bodybuilders negotiate normative femininity in competitive bodybuilding. *Women's Studies Quarterly, 33*(1–2), 134–149.

Breivik, G., Hanstad, D. V., & Loland, S. (2009). Attitudes towards the use of performance-enhancing substances and body modification techniques: A comparison between elite athletes and the general population. *Sport in Society: Cultures, Commerce, Media, Politics, 12*(6), 737–754.

Bunsell, T. (2013). *Strong and hard women: An ethnography of female bodybuilding.* London: Routledge.

Butler, J. (1990). *Gender trouble: Feminism and the subversion of identity.* London: Routledge.

Butler, J. (1993). *Bodies that matter: On the discursive limits of "sex"*. London: Routledge.

Butler, J. (2004). *Undoing gender*. New York: Routledge.

Christiansen, A. V. (2018). *Motionsdoping: Styrketræning, identitet og kultur* [Recreational doping: Strength training, identity and culture]. Aarhus, Denmark: Aarhus Universitetsforlag.

Denham, B. E. (2008). Masculinities in hardcore bodybuilding. *Men and Masculinities, 11*(2), 234–242.

Evans-Brown, M., & McVeigh, J. (2009). Anabolic steroid use in the general population of the United Kingdom. In V. Møller, M. McNamee, & P. Dimeo (Eds.), *Elite sport, doping and public health* (pp. 75–97). Odense, Denmark: University Press of Southern Denmark.

Fair, J. D. (1999). *Muscletown USA: Bob Hoffman and the manly culture of York Barbell*. University Park: Pennsylvania State University Press.

Field, A., Austin, S., Camargo, C., Taylor, C. B., Striegel-Moore, R. H., Loud, K. J. & Colditz, G. A. (2005). Exposure to the mass media, body shape concerns, and use of supplements to improve weight and shape among male and female adolescents. *Pediatrics, 116*(2), 214–220.

Griffet, J. (2000). The path chosen by female bodybuilders: A tentative interpretation. *Sociology of Sport Journal, 17*, 130–150.

Grogan, S. (2006). Body image and health: Contemporary perspectives. *Journal of Health Psychology, 11*(4), 523–530.

Grogan, S., Evans, R., Wright, S., & Hunter, G. (2004). Femininity and muscularity: Accounts of seven women body builders. *Journal of Gender Studies, 13*(1), 49–61.

Haraway, D. (1990). A Manifesto for cyborgs: Science, technology and socialist feminism in the 1980's. In L. J. Nicholson (Ed.), *Feminism/postmodernism*. London: Routledge.

Hill Collins, P. (2000). *Black feminist thought: Knowledge, consciousness, and the politics of empowerment* (2nd ed.). New York, NY: Routledge.

IFBB. (2018). *Our disciplines*. Retrieved March 10, 2018, from https://ifbb.com/our-disciplines/.

Jespersen, M. R. (2012). "Definitely not for women": An online community's reflections on women's use of performance enhancing drugs. In J. Tolleneer, S. Sterckx, & P. Bonte (Eds.), *Athletic enhancement, human nature and ethics: Threats and opportunities of doping technologies* (pp. 201–218). Dordrecht, The Netherlands: Springer.

Klein, A. (1993). *Little big men: Bodybuilding, subculture and gender construction*. New York: State University of New York Press.

Lindsay, C. (1996). Bodybuilding: A postmodern freak show. In R. G. Thomson (Ed.), *Freakery: Cultural spectacles of the extraordinary body*. New York: New York University Press.

Liokaftos, D. (2018). Natural bodybuilding: An account of its emergence and development as competition sport. *International Review for the Sociology of Sports* (Online), 1–18.

Malcolm, N. L. (2000). Constructing female athleticism: A study of girls' recreational softball. *American Behavioral Scientist, 46*(10), 1304–1387.

McGrath, S., & Chananie-Hill, R. (2009). 'Big Freaky-Looking Women': Normalizing gender transgression through bodybuilding. *Sociology of Sport Journal, 26,* 235–254.

Monaghan, L. (2001). *Bodybuilding, drugs and risk: Health, risk and society*. New York: Routledge.

Monaghan, L. F. (2012). Accounting for illicit steroid use: Bodybuilders' justifications. In A. Locks & N. Richardson (Eds.), *Critical readings in bodybuilding* (pp. 73–90). New York, NY: Routledge.

Muller, S., Gorrow, T. R., & Schneider, S. R. (2009). Enhancing appearance and sports performance: Are female collegiate athletes behaving more like males? *Journal of American College Health, 57*(5), 513–520.

Richardson, N. (2008). Flex-rated! Female bodybuilding: Feminist resistance or erotic spectacle? *Journal of Gender Studies, 17*(4), 289–301.

Roussel, P., Monaghan, L., Javerlhiac, S., & Yondre, F. (2010). The metamorphosis of female bodybuilders: Judging a paroxysmal body? *International Review for the Sociology of Sport, 45*(1), 103–109.

Sagoe, D., Andreassen, C. S., & Pallesen, S. (2014). The aetiology and trajectory of anabolic-androgenic steroid use initiation: A systematic review and synthesis of qualitative research. *Substance Abuse Treatment, Prevention, and Policy, 9,* 1–14. https://doi.org/10.1186/1747-597x-9-27.

Sassatelli, R. (2010). *Fitness culture: Gyms and the commercialisation of discipline and fun*. Houndmills, UK: Palgrave Macmillan.

Smith, A. C. T., & Stewart, B. (2012). Body perceptions and health behaviors in an online bodybuilding community. *Qualitative Health Research, 22*(7), 971–985.

The Swedish Doping Act. (1991:1969). *Dopningslagen*. Stockholm, Sweden: Svensk författningssamling SFS.

Thualagant, N. (2012). The conceptualization of fitness doping and its limitations. *Sport in society: Cultures, commerce, media, politics, 15*(3), 409–419.

Van Hout, M. C., & Hearne, E. (2016). Netnography of female use of the synthetic growth hormone CJC-1295: Pulses and potions. *Substance Use and Misuse, 51*(1), 73–84.

Part IV

Conclusions

9

Trajectories and the New Doping Demography

Introduction

At the beginning of this concluding chapter, a brief reminder regarding the historical development of gym culture and fitness doping is in place. As argued, the cultural history of fitness doping is clearly one of transforming cultures, ideals, lifestyles, and bodies. It is also a history of the development of contemporary sport and of gender. Originally, fitness doping was mainly connected to bodybuilding. With roots from the early twentieth century, the classical bodybuilding body was promoted in alliance with the development of *physical culture* and given shape in the gym. For the most part, it was a male body being formed, which fit nicely into a national culture that was valorizing masculinity, discipline, and nationalism. Different techniques for developing bodies and building muscles, including the use of fitness doping, were initially understood as part of a scientific approach to the body and the development of an industrial society. Consequently, during the 1940s and 1950s, use of performance- and image-enhancing drugs (PIEDs) was not particularly problematized, but rather seen as connected to the development of modern medicine,

© The Author(s) 2020
J. Andreasson and T. Johansson, *Fitness Doping*,
https://doi.org/10.1007/978-3-030-22105-8_9

sport, scientific management and more broadly also to modernity and ideas about how to build a modern society.

During the 1970s and 1980s, bodybuilding, as well as gym and fitness culture in general, underwent remarkable transformations. Bodybuilding came to be seen as something of a postmodern spectacle. The bodies produced through drug use practices now began to represent something extreme, subcultural, and the desire to expand the limits of what was achievable in terms of transforming human bodies and reaching the genetic maximum. Ideals connected to modernity and industrialization were thus gradually replaced by something else, perhaps a pastiche. Interestingly, this development also coincides with the development of anti-doping work conducted in the context of organized elite sport, in general, and establishment of the WADA, in particular. Thus, it is reasonable to assume that the notion of maintaining fair play in sport through anti-doping efforts also came to influence people's perceptions and the cultural structuration of the meaning of fitness doping.

The idea of fair play and drug-free sports has had a certain impact on bodybuilding and fitness athletics, but the picture is more complex. When bodybuilding developed, so did the desire to create fantastic bodies and transgress all existing boundaries through the use of PIEDs, new training techniques and diets. There are also many descriptions of how the need for refined drugs and hormones during this period pushed bodybuilding into the 'dark.' Furthermore, the costs associated with the drugs and the lifestyle of a bodybuilder often forced competitors to, for example, commit illegal acts or hustle (Klein, 1993). The image of a vibrant subcultural phenomenon was thus reinforced in the 1970s and 1980s, only to be pushed underground more or less involuntarily in the 1990s. Fitness culture 'entered the scene' of shaping bodies.

Since the 1990s, the development of gym and fitness culture has been tremendous. In this book, the growth, expansion and commercialization of gym culture and the cultural transformation of fit bodies have been conceptualized in terms of a *fitness revolution*. Included in this cultural revolution and structural transformation process is a strong connection between what can be considered more subcultural developments of body ideals, drug use practices and gender configurations, and the development of training techniques, body ideals, and practices that have promoted a more dynamic, flexible and gender-inclusive body and health culture. As noted, the gradual separation between drugs associated with bodybuilding culture and fitness, however, does not mean these phenomena have turned into two different, separate activities and lifestyles. Rather, these two conceptions of exercise and lifestyle have partly become disconnected and partly increasingly dependent on each other. Thus, contemporary perspectives on fitness doping should be understood as a composition of various simultaneous tendencies, such as the general and widespread performance culture, the commercialization of beauty, the increased interest in health and fitness, and the development of modern medicine, as well as the possibilities to use licit or illicit substances to change the human (subcultural) body. It is within the context of this culture in transformation, or with the help of this cultural elixir and all its complexities, that we have aimed to do two things in this book. First, we have tried to investigate and discuss different processes through which a person becomes a fitness doper. In doing so, we have attempted to, second, say something relevant about the impact this cultural development has had on the gendering and gender politics attached to the practice and the fitness doping demography.

Staying true to the overall aims of the book, in the remainder of this chapter we develop our line of reasoning concerning the cultural development of gym and fitness and synthesize its impact on fitness doping trajectories. We also pick up on some central discussions concerning gendered understandings of fitness doping and conclude our thoughts on a fitness doping demography in transition. The chapter also includes a discussion on health and lifestyles, the significance of online communities and an argument regarding how the so-called subcultural use of doping can be understood theoretically. Concerning the latter, we look in particular at the relationship between subcultural relations and belongings and broader contemporary societal developments.

Doping Trajectories

Although the use of doping in gym and fitness environments has been considered a public health issue internationally for quite some time, there is surprisingly little scholarship on fitness doping trajectories (Christiansen, Schmidt Vinter, & Liokaftos, 2016; McNamee et al., 2014; McVeigh, Bates & Chandler, 2015). Whereas many existing models on doping initiation focus on psychological, psychiatric and, thus, individual explanations, in this book we have aimed at taking a broader range of approaches when trying to understand diverse trajectories. Furthermore, we have tried not to focus solely on doping use in relation to strength training and bodybuilding, an area traditionally dominated by young men, but also analyzed how use is understood by women and people engaged in a variety of training forms in the gym and fitness context. Our findings confirm the notion that there are many ways to enter and exit a subcultural space, where doping is viewed as part of a certain lifestyle.

Fitness doping trajectories—that is, the processes involved when a person is becoming and unbecoming a fitness doper—need to be understood on different, but intersecting levels. *First,* we have the individual and psychological level, which has been studied by a great number of scholars. Here we find a large body of literature in which use is, and has been, discussed in relation to individual characteristics, upbringing, relationships to parents (in particular fathers), sporting background, potential youth criminality, a person's sense of self-worth, body issues, self-image, and other psychological variables. Individual features—sometimes discursively connected to more or less pathological and psychiatric identifications (such as Megarexi, the Adonis complex and later Orthorexia)—have had a huge impact on the field. Thus, subjective meanings have largely been understood as formative of men's and women's potential engagement in and attitudes toward drug use practices, as well as their perceptions of the associated health risks (Pope, Phillips & Olivardia, 2002). Some scholars have also created models intended to help in predicting potential users. In doing so, they have contributed to confusion regarding what scientific claims can reasonably be made based on usually small samples and unsystematic studies. Others have been more modest and reasonable in their claims, and instead developed typologies that can be used as heuristic tools for understanding people's initiation into drug use. For instance, Christiansen et al. (2016) created a typology to help us understand the various motives underlying and the distinct and characteristic approaches to fitness doping. Focusing on male steroid users, they describe *the expert type, the well-being type, the YOLO type,* and *the athlete type.*

Although these types and the typology have a bearing on the empirical findings and have contributed greatly to our understanding of individual motives and trajectories, some concerns can be raised regarding the risks associated with over-diagnosing. When compiling this literature, there is a tendency to approach concepts, such as identity and self, as isolated phenomena, rather than as actions that are performed or done in relation to social encounters, contexts and cultural affiliations. Therefore, in this book, we have not lingered on psychologically informed models and labels. Instead, trajectories have been understood as messier, more non-linear and more contingent, and as a part of a more general sociocultural development, which has greatly impacted people's ways of understanding and relating to the body and self, even outside the sphere of gym and fitness culture.

Second, becoming part of a specific subcultural milieu also entails developing certain values, attitudes, and behaviors. Entering into this subcultural space—where much of everyday life revolves around muscles, training schedules, diet, a strict lifestyle, and fitness doping—also means renegotiating and eventually also reconceptualizing the individual's way of approaching and understanding the world at large. This leads to, among other things, a growing distance and cleavage between the individual and his/her old friends. There are manifold ways to describe these distancing processes—processes through which the individual, by different means and both online and offline, legitimizes and normalizes drug use, particularly as part of a lifestyle-forming practice. Entering into to the subcultural space of drug use also entails making new connections and friends, while simultaneously (perhaps) leaving other relationships behind. These processes have more or less solely been discussed in relation to homosocial subcultural belongings with male connotations (Christiansen, 2018; Klein, 1993; Monaghan, 2001, 2012). In the book, we have also tried to show how gym and fitness culture has expanded and has in some ways, not least in terms of its spatiality, become more gender inclusive. Consequently, there are strong reasons to reconceptualize the gendering of fitness doping trajectories. Approaching gym and fitness culture, in general, and fitness doping, in particular, as a phenomenon that reaches well beyond male muscle building practices also requires that we rethink how drug use is understood in relation to gender. We will return to this discussion in a while.

Third, when approaching fitness doping trajectories, we have suggested that it is vital to not only include the significance of gym and fitness culture, but also to position this development in the broader societal context of a Western performance-oriented, individualized, and medicalized society (Conrad, 2007). Thualagant (2012), for example, uses the concept of a *doped society*, describing a performance-culture-based society that encourages its inhabitants to strive for the right body. In order to optimize their human capital, modern individuals are prepared to take all necessary measures, one of which may be doping. The process involved in the cultural commercialization of health within the fitness industry can certainly be seen as a positive development, as promoting physical exercise and healthy eating habits helps prevent disease, at least to some extent. Nevertheless, it has also increasingly turned the body and its appearance into important markers of how healthy or successful a person is or is deemed to be.

Following these lines of thought, we have argued that—depending on how far individuals are prepared to go to reach their goals and push their body projects forward and create something desirable—some will choose to take drugs while others will be satisfied with 'only' exposing their bodies to different training regimes. Conceptualizing fitness doping trajectories in this way shows that they could be understood as activities performed along a continuum of cultural and societal conformity, rather than as actions representing societal abnormality. This way of reasoning highlights how vital corporeal investments/results can be to the construction of subjectivity in an individualized society, which of course affects people's propensity to engage in drug use practices. We argue that it can also help revitalize ongoing discussions on so-called exit processes and trajectories leading away from fitness doping, a topic that is still under-researched.

Challenging Gender and the Internet

The willingness to perform, to focus on the body's *functions, physiology and capacity*, can certainly be seen as a paradigmatic account that is idealized in narratives on fitness doping. As such, these narratives can be situated in and understood as a fairly stable part of a hegemonic masculine construction (Connell, 1995; Connell & Messerschmidt, 2005). Historically, masculinity has been constituted as something to be accomplished and performed, especially with the help of bulging muscles. However, within an individualized fitness culture, this celebrated and performance-oriented lifestyle seems to be entwined with a strong passion for bodily esthetics—for beautiful, commercialized, and slender bodies, all of which focus on the *appearance* of the body (Smith Maguire, 2008)—and connected to the notion of emphasized femininity. This cultural development of individualization, performance, and appearance creates cultural ambiguity that can be used as a window through which we can analyze different transformations and understandings of gender, and how they are manifested on the fit and potentially doped body in contemporary society, both in the context of online communication and away from keyboard.

Although fitness doping still can be understood in terms of hegemonic patterns—where men dominate the scene and set the agenda for fitness doping—our results point to a development in which women have gradually become integrated into the community of PIED users. Contesting the alliance between masculinity and fitness doping, introducing women as active and competent doping users, and exploring the ongoing gender-bending present in fitness culture indicate, for example, that women are not to the same extent dependent on men to obtain drug reports. There is also an increasing amount of knowledge, not only aimed at but also developed by and for women, on the Internet. Thus, not only has the culture of fitness expanded in relation to gender, but owing to the technological push, we have also seen the emergence of a new globalized arena for fitness doping. Since introduced, social media and different Internet forums have become an intrinsic, integrated part of gym and fitness and a new *self-help culture* where one can engage both in the manifestation/construction of body ideals and lifestyles and in doping. The online way of closing in on, and potentially entering into, the doping experience exists in a context that is not bound by national laws, policies, or prevention strategies. Naturally, this has had a great impact on the face of fitness doping. Face-to-face encounters have partly been replaced with Internet chat groups or with other types of social media-based interactions where perfect bodies (both male and female) are visualized and celebrated. Consequently, huge numbers of interactions are taking place on the Internet, and there is no longer a need for a specific mentor or advisor. Instead, online communications facilitate the availability of myriad voices, guiding new users—women and men, young and old—into the practices. In a certain sense, what is happening here is that new kinds of learning processes are being developed on the Internet. In addition to this development, it has become more difficult to distinguish between the 'authentic' subculture, with masculine connotations, and the more general, transitional processes of becoming involved in a physical culture, where a disciplined lifestyle is combined with using certain drugs and hormones. We live in a culture where the fit bodies of men and women are constantly being put on display and commercialized, for example, on social media. This development also presents a huge challenge to subcultural theories and youth cultural approaches to fitness culture, in general, and fitness doping, in particular.

Naturally, the new ethno-pharmacological culture on the Internet comes with certain risks and dangers. On the one hand, mentors and advice are easily available on the various chat groups and forums. On the other, there is a minimum of control and risk analysis. The subcultural phenomenon of bodybuilding and its at times naive celebration of PIEDs are, in a certain sense, being brought closer to 'ordinary people.' This is also one of the key mechanisms underlying what we have called fitness doping. The tremendous development of both gym and fitness culture and the Internet has in a sense brought subcultural and more general cultural phenomena together. In this intermixture of different perspectives on training schedules, diets, gender, drugs, and body ideals, the new fitness doping phenomenon and demography are evolving and taking shape.

The spatiality and the gendered dimensions of fitness doping demographics are set in motion. This development can also be read as part of the normalization of fitness doping. Following in the wake of the technological push, and as it becomes clear that fitness doping use among the general population is a growing phenomenon, new ways of understanding this issue need to be brought to the fore. Looking at preventative measures directed at fitness dopers, anti-doping work, although meant to be random, still largely employs muscle profiling when testing (men) at gyms (van de Ven & Mulrooney, 2016). As we have discussed, this means that female fitness doping has largely escaped both scholarly attention and preventative anti-doping work.

To meet these changes in the gendering and development of a new fitness doping demography, we would like to suggest a re-articulation of hegemonic masculinity, breaking with Connell's notion that hegemonic masculinity is always defined in opposition to 'emphasized femininity.' This is a term chosen deliberately to fix femininity—even in theory—in a position that is always subordinate to masculinity (Connell & Messerschmidt, 2005). If we break this connection, we may well argue that what hegemonic masculinity represents is not a discourse that ultimately always serves to subjugate women/femininity. What we have to break with then is also the notion that all forms of hegemony are equally bad and that the ultimate goal of any emancipatory struggle must be to do away with hegemony. What we need to do is to try to disentangle the notion of hegemony from its taken-for-granted connection to a specific form of masculinity and femininity (Johansson & Ottemo, 2015). If we are able to do so, we can reconceptualize fitness doping and understand it less in terms of stereotypical and marginalized masculinities and more in terms of issues of health and the development of certain lifestyles. We discuss this further in the next section.

Health and Lifestyles

The fitness industry has helped establish strong links between certain very strict and disciplined body ideals and the notion of a healthy lifestyle. In this context, obesity and overweight signal poor health, an unhealthy lifestyle and, to a certain extent, even personality flaws. The question is what impact the increasing market for PIEDs, plastic surgery, and sophisticated body modification techniques will have on people's perceptions of health and morality. As we have touched on, it is possible to talk about a new fitness doping demography in which not only the gendered dimensions of drug use are reconceptualized, but also how use is connected to, for example, aging. What we can discern from our material is also how our participants negotiate and find their own ways of puzzling together a 'healthy lifestyle' with using certain amounts of hormones and steroids.

This increasing experimentation with different substances is part of a new ethno-pharmacology (developed within even larger processes of medicalization in society), which is a stock of knowledge comprising: a taxonomy of different steroids, theories of usage, methods of administration, awareness of different side effects, and strategies to avoid them (Monaghan, 2001). On the one hand, this way of consecrating fitness doping is an important part of the construction of a subcultural space. For instance, many bodybuilders and fitness competitors view drug use as a legitimate means of attaining a subculturally prescribed goal. On the other hand, although the individuals who give others advice, for example, through an Internet community, seem to be knowledgeable and well informed, our information on how these people obtained their knowledge is limited. Although many narratives presented here indicate that users are more or less aware of the risks involved in using PIEDs, some also tend to downplay these risks and develop their own (subcultural) position. We can see, for example, a tendency to argue that other people use alcohol, spend too much time in front of the television, and eat bad food, and that it is much better to embrace a healthy lifestyle, combined with PIED use. This way of calculating the risks involved, and of elaborating *private theories* on how different aspects of fitness doping may become part of a healthy lifestyle, is also very characteristic of a subcultural symbolic space.

The logics of the subcultural space are often somewhat twisted and queer. This 'space' often stretches from face-to-face interactions in certain demarcated social and cultural contexts to a diversity of Internet forums, blogs, and chat groups. Individuals within this space develop a certain way of framing, talking about and perceiving the practices necessary to develop the ideal body. Not infrequently, these ways of framing and thinking about training regimes, diets, and steroids are at odds with the legal system and general perceptions of health and risks in society at large.

What we see today is, perhaps, a *new phase* in the historical development of views on fitness doping in the context of gym and fitness culture (see Chapter 2). Although the short-term (side) effects of PIEDs have been known for decades, and evidence regarding the long-term health effects and consequences are now beginning to accumulate (Christiansen et al., 2016), critics of the strict anti-doping policies around the world still argue that there is a lack of evidence concerning the negative effects of human growth hormones and sometimes even steroids. They believe that because PIEDs have not been subject to critical investigations, they have come to be defined and seen as detrimental to users' health. Critics of the anti-doping position are gradually gaining ground, arguing that harm-free drugs may be manufactured in the future. In order for anti-doping work to continue, it will probably be necessary to elaborate new arguments in relation to (public) health, and to defend, for example, the intrinsic values of sport and the ethical ideas of natural bodybuilding.

Merging Subculture and Common Culture

In this book, we have elaborated on the relation between subcultures and what we have called common culture or mainstream culture. Clearly, it is not particularly difficult to discern, describe and analyze subcultural formations in fitness culture. However, trying to define mainstream or common culture is more difficult and challenging. It may be that there are no clear and useful definitions of what is common. However, using this distinction, we have tried to come closer to understanding the dynamic and changing relation between a body culture that challenges our understanding of what is a 'normal' body and lifestyle and a more normalized, everyday understanding of the human body. Nearing the end of the book, we will try to elaborate a bit more on this conceptual pair and to extend it, with a view to trying to interpret and understand some of the results presented.

Using Homi Bhaba's (1994) concept of a *third space*, it is possible to explore the relation between these two conceptual arenas. The concept of a third space originates in a postcolonial perspective and aims at conceptualizing *hybrid identities* in a changing world. Bhaba is influenced by linguistics and post-structural language theories, but he extends these theories, applying them to culture.

It is that Third Space, though unrepresentable in itself, which constitutes the discursive conditions of enunciation that ensures that the meaning and symbols of culture have no primordial unity or fixity; that even the same signs can be appropriated, translated, rehistoricized and read anew. (Bhaba, 1994, p. 55)

In the context of our study, using the concept of a *third space* would suggest a somewhat different application. As we have seen, fitness doping is not a matter of either-or, but rather both-and. Many of the participants who have contributed their stories and experiences have talked about how they both try to fit into society, living a largely ordinary life, but at the same time participate in a highly distinct and exclusive subcultural space, where extraordinary bodies are sculptured and created. Trying to balance between being part of society and part of a specific subculture is clearly demanding. It seems like many of our participants are searching for a way to switch between different lifestyles, and thus to achieve a certain balance between their, in one sense, dual identities. Within the Third Space, fitness dopers operate and negotiate the meaning of the drugs, and their use is rationalized, legitimized, and understood as a necessary part of a certain lifestyle. Within this space, drug use is also challenged through social interaction and cultural encounters. Using this concept as an analytical prism through which we can understand fitness doping in transition, we aspire to get closer to what is actually taking place in many of our participants' lives.

In the book, we have investigated and explored what we have called a *new fitness doping demography*. Using the concept of a third space, we wish to focus on *the intermediary area*—an area in between subcultural spaces and society at large. In particular, we have tried to explore areas of overlap and intermixtures between what are regarded as extreme bodies and sports, and societal and preferred ways of idealizing and talking about healthy and 'perfect' bodies. This way of approaching the phenomenon blurs to some extent the borderlines between acceptable and illegitimate methods of constructing fitness bodies. This quite recent development raises new questions about prevention and social work. It also challenges how we navigate in a changing world, especially in a world where acceleration processes and technological innovations affect how we look at bodies, health, and risks.

Final Remarks—Issues and Controversies

There are reasons to suspect that we are entering an era in gym and fitness culture, as well as in society in large, in which it is possible to talk about a new fitness doping geography and demography. During its historical development, this culture of fit bodies has transformed into a mass leisure activity, and having gym membership is largely considered, at least in the West, a must for anyone who wishes to pursue a decent body. As a cultural phenomenon of shaping bodies, we are definitely no longer bound to subcultural, homosocial basement facilities where bodybuilders invest a great deal of time and commitment, and for that matter drug use practices, to create the perfect body. Instead, we have a wide variety of premises ranging from classical bodybuilding gyms to luxury spas. Obviously, there is a movement toward cultural, spatial, and *architectural gentrification*. To this end, the cultural geography and demography of the gym have changed, broadening tremendously within a relatively short period of time. Paradoxically, however, along with this process of mainstreaming gym and fitness culture, thoughts about doping have endured, and although bodybuilders are still often exposed to negative muscle profiling, there are strong indications of a more complex doping demography.

We have argued not only for the need to contest and possibly deconstruct doping use as a phenomenon that can neatly be tied to either elite competitive bodybuilders or athletes within the formally governed elite sport context, but also for an analysis of how the values and ideals acquired through youth sport participation may or may not be transferred to the context of gym and fitness culture (Brennan, Wells, & van Hout, 2017). Thus, when developing prevention strategies, the nexus between doping in sport and fitness doping and health promotion strategies needs to be taken into consideration. Following this line of thought, and talking about cultural contexts, we further argue for the need to investigate the negotiations of fitness doping taking place at the intersection between subcultural affiliations/spaces and mainstream perceptions of living an ordinary (read 'normal') life. As we have shown, processes of (un)becoming a fitness doper are anything but linear, and thus, they need to be understood in relation to sociocultural belonging and ongoing negotiations of the individual's sense of self, gender, health, and family responsibilities.

References

Bhaba, H. (1994). *The location of culture.* London: Routledge.

Brennan, R., Wells, J., & van Hout, M. C. (2017). The injecting use of image and performance-enhancing drugs (IPED) in the general population: A systematic review. *Health and Social Care in the Community, 25*(5), 1459–1531.

Christiansen, A. V. (2018). *Motionsdoping. Styrketræning, identitet og kultur* [Recreational doping: Strength training, identity and culture]. Aarhus, Denmark: Aarhus Universitetsforlag.

Christiansen, A. V., Schmidt Vinther, A., & Liokaftos, D. (2016). Outline of a typology of men's use of anabolic androgenic steroids in fitness and strength training environments. *Drugs: Education, Prevention and Policy,* https://doi.org/10.1080/09687637.2016.1231173.

Connell, R. W. (1995). *Masculinities.* Cambridge: Polity Press.

Connell, R. W., & Messerschmidt, J. W. (2005). Hegemonic masculinity: Rethinking the concept. *Gender & Society, 19,* 829–859.

Conrad, P. (2007). *The medicalization of society: On the transformation of human conditions into treatable disorders.* Baltimore, MD: Johns Hopkins University Press.

Johansson, T., & Ottemo, A. (2015). Ruptures in hegemonic masculinity: The dialectic between ideology and utopia. *Journal of Gender Studies, 24*(2), 192–206.

Klein, A. (1993). *Little big men: Bodybuilding, subculture and gender construction.* New York: State University of New York Press.

McNamee, M., Backhouse, S. H., Defoort, Y., Parkinson, A., Sauer, M., & Collins, C. (2014). *Study on doping prevention: A map of legal, regulatory and prevention practice provisions in EU 28.* Luxembourg. Retrieved from http://www.studyondopingprevention.eu/.

McVeigh, J., Bates, G., & Chandler, M. (2015). *Steroids and image enhancing drugs—2014 survey results.* Retrieved from http://www.ipedinfo.co.uk/resources/downloads/SIEDs%20Survey%20report%202014%20FINAL.pdf.

Monaghan, L. F. (2001). *Bodybuilding, drugs and risk: Health, risk and society.* New York: Routledge.

Monaghan, L. F. (2012). Accounting for illicit steroid use: Bodybuilders' justifications. In A. Locks & N. Richardson (Red.), *Critical readings in bodybuilding.* New York: Routledge.

Pope, H. G., Phillips, K. A., & Olivardia, R. (2002). *The adonis complex: How to identify, treat, and prevent body obsession in men and boys.* New York, NY: Simon & Schuster.

Smith Maguire, J. (2008). *Fit for consumption: Sociology and the business of fitness.* London and New York: Routledge.

Thualagant, N. (2012). The conceptualization of fitness doping and its limitations. *Sport in Society: Cultures, Commerce, Media, Politics, 15*(3), 409–419.

van de Ven, K., & Mulrooney, K. (2016). How private gyms work to keep their members from doping. *The Conversation.* Retrieved January 5, 2019, from https://www.businessinsider.com/private-gyms-members-doping-2016-12?r=US&IR=T&IR=T.

10

Research Design and Methodological Considerations

Introduction

Fitness Doping: Trajectories, Gender, Bodies and Health is the outcome of a joint collaboration in which we, Jesper Andreasson and Thomas Johansson, have carried out studies on fitness doping during the period 2014 to 2019. But we actually began this work even earlier, as the book is part of a larger ethnographical 'umbrella' project in which different aspects of gym and fitness culture have been analyzed over some ten years. Using qualitative measures, we have previously taken part in the everyday lives of, for example, personal trainers, fitness professionals, gym owners, and dedicated gym-goers. We have also previously published two books—*The Global Gym: Gender, Health and Pedagogies* (2014) and *Extreme Sports, Extreme Bodies: Gender, Identities and Bodies in Motion* (2019)—with Palgrave Macmillan. In this sense, this book on fitness doping should be understood as the third and final part of a puzzle we have tried to complete over a number of years, analyzing and writing about the development of gym and fitness culture and its effects on the human body, gender ideals, and health, among other issues.

© The Author(s) 2020
J. Andreasson and T. Johansson, *Fitness Doping*,
https://doi.org/10.1007/978-3-030-22105-8_10

Although part of a larger puzzle, for this book we have relied solely on data from fitness doping users. Taking an ethnographic approach to the research, we have, as stated previously, attempted to grasp various aspects of fitness doping in the chapters, and in this final chapter, we summarize the method and methodology used in completing the book. Basically, the book builds on data gathered using a qualitative mixed method approach, consisting of qualitative biographical interviews, observations, Internet material, and an overall ethnographic approach to the research (Fangen, 2005; Hammersley & Atkinson, 1995).

Obviously, conducting ethnographic research can mean many things. Hammersley and Atkinson (1995) describe ethnography not just as a method, but rather as a collection of methods with which the researcher can—in different ways and more or less openly—participate in the everyday lives of others (see also Fangen, 2005; Gratton & Jones, 2004). This open and wide-ranging definition of research in the social sciences is close to the methodological starting point of the research on which this book is based. We have used various methods to establish relationships with people operating within the gym and fitness context who have experiences of using performance- and image-enhancing drugs (PIEDs). Our ambition has been to describe, both theoretically and empirically, their everyday lives and perspectives. As a consequence of this methodological and epistemological position, we have also considered it counterproductive to try to define boundaries between ethnography and other qualitative, empirically intimate, research methods. Instead, regarding epistemology, we understand ethnography not primarily as a method, but rather, as Anderson-Levitt (2006) argues, as a philosophy of research. Our belief is that when the aim is to investigate and understand human settings, in general, and fitness doping trajectories, in particular, a relational epistemology is preferable. The scope of data collection strategies and our ethnographic approach should thus be understood as a form of methodological triangulation intended to expose: 'unique differences or meaningful information that may have remained undiscovered with the use of only one approach or data collection technique in the study' (Thurmond, 2001, p. 255).

Although a variety of approaches to data collection has been utilized, the book mainly derives from two somewhat separate projects or contexts of research. *First*, we have a longitudinal ethnographic study in which drug users have been interviewed and observed in everyday life. *Second*, we have a netnographic study in which data from online communications have been gathered. These two datasets or sub-projects obviously differ in some ways, which is the reason they are presented and discussed separately below. However, when writing the book, the data have largely been treated and understood as tightly interwoven in the different chapters and guided by our shared, overall aim, as formulated in Chapter 1.

This chapter is structured as follows. Next, we explain the method and methodology for the longitudinal ethnographic study we conducted. We touch upon issues such as sampling, interviews and observation, and how the gathered data have been analyzed. Thereafter follows a section in which we explain how the netnographic study was designed and how online communications have been treated analytically. Both of these sections also include a discussion on research ethics. Finally, the chapter ends with some comments on the national comparative study presented in Chapter 3, which was written by Jesper Andreasson and April Dawn Henning, at the University of Stirling. Because this study falls partly outside the joint collaboration between us, Jesper Andreasson, and Thomas Johansson, it has a separate methodological section.

Longitudinal Ethnographic Study

The main corpus of data used for this book derives from a longitudinal ethnographical study, which typically entailed interviews, informal conversations, and observations in the environments where the participating fitness dopers performed and interacted in their everyday life. Results from this study/project have mainly been used in Chapters 4, 5, 7, and 8, and to some extent also in Chapter 3.

Because possession and use of PIEDs is criminalized in Sweden, where most of the data have been gathered, getting in contact with and gaining the trust of PIED users were challenging. Initially, various strategies were used to identify and approach potential participants. *First*, certain organizations were helpful. For example, a Swedish organization that helps ex-convicts reintegrate into society (KRIS) and Sweden's 'anti-doping hotline' (*Dopingjouren*) assisted and provided some contacts. KRIS is an association started by ex-criminals that aims to help people who have been released from prison stay away from crime and drugs, offering them an honest and drug-free social network. The Anti-Doping Hot-Line is a Swedish nation-wide telephone consulting service, which one can call anonymously with questions about doping. The service of the Anti-Doping Hot-Line is funded by the Ministry of Health and Social Affairs and the Ministry of Culture. *Second*, the Swedish fitness magazine *Body* was approached and agreed to letting a description of the research project appear on their Web site. This magazine is probably the most iconic and well-known medium on the Swedish bodybuilding scene. Bodybuilders and fitness competitors are regularly pictured and interviewed there, sharing their training advice and more (see, https://www.body.se/). A few participants were recruited using this strategy. *Third*, additional contacts were established through Jesper's participation in a community project working to spread knowledge about PIEDs in local schools, sports, and fitness centers. The most important source, however, was existing participants, who provided additional contacts for a second selection stage, using a respondent-driven sample or snowball-sampling (Agar, 1996; Lalander, 2003; Salganik & Heckathorn, 2004).

One important aim of the sampling was to ensure variation among the participants regarding their training objectives, age, extent of PIED experience, training routine, and ways of looking at the body and gender. As our network of participants grew, we were also able to discuss our sampling with key participants, thus directing the recruitment process toward this ambition. A total of 31 participants (24 men, 7 women) contributed their stories. Most have been interviewed on more than one occasion, a total of 65 formal interviews were conducted and an estimated 40 days were spent on observations, including numerous informal conversations (Fangen, 2005). A majority of the participants were between 25 and 35 years old during the study period. The oldest person interviewed was 64, and the youngest 19 when recruited. All interviews, which were between one to four hours in length, have been audio-recorded and transcribed verbatim.

As regards the interviews, they were conducted using a biographical and narrative approach (Hallqvist & Hydén, 2012; Merill & West, 2009; Shamir, Daya-Horesh, & Adler, 2005). We were interested in following different social and cultural trajectories through storytelling and the ordering of important life events. In general, the first interview was semi-structured in the sense that the questions dealt with specific themes (such as the participant's socioeconomic background, fitness doping experience, health, gender and, of course, processes of becoming a user of fitness doping). Thus, we asked the participants how their first contact with doping manifested itself and how they viewed their drug use. We also asked them how they understood drug use in relation to the body, sense of self, gender, friends and family, and doping prevention, among other issues. Follow-up interviews were usually less structured and designed to elicit more detailed descriptions and transitional processes/perspectives on the participant's drug use. Of relevance here was the prolonged period in which the participants were involved in the project (approximately five years), which allowed us to capture their fitness doping trajectories. Hence, the narratives provided detailed descriptions not only of why the participants engaged in the practice, but also why some of them later chose to unbecome fitness doping users.

In addition, to establish relationships of trust and be able to challenge/validate the interview data, when possible we followed the participants in their everyday life—participating, for example, in various training situations. Fieldwork was carried out using direct observation. We took notes during or after an interaction and summed up our notes at the end of the research day. The advantage of using 'direct' observations is that being present 'when and where it happens' can yield knowledge that is different from and complementary to the information provided in an interview situation, for example. The observations gave us an opportunity to contextualize the verbal. Conducting observations was also beneficial because it enabled us to investigate various aspects of the research settings that might otherwise have been forgotten or perceived as trivial by the participants. This constituted an attempt to capture what Giddens (1986) has termed practical knowledge, which refers to incorporated physical know-how that guides the individual. Because this knowledge is embodied, it most often remains unspoken and, therefore, difficult to detect through interviews alone (Pink, 2009).

Within ethnography, data collection does not occur in isolation from data analysis (Hammersley & Atkinson, 1995). Using our verbatim transcripts and observational notes, we continuously read our empirical material and made theoretically informed notes during this process. Our ambition was to identify shared understandings and similar phrases in the data and to so to speak validate our analytical ideas when conducting new interviews and observations. To us, this type of analysis, combined with a multitude of empirical settings and sources, provided rich ground on which to produce nuanced *thick descriptions* (Geertz, 1973) of fitness dopers. Furthermore, because doping trajectories are generated in social interaction, our analysis needed to be able to capture movements and changes over time, as well as complexities and contradictions. One of our reasons for following the participants ethnographically over time was to be able to analyze both situational aspects and alterations. Back (2012a, 2012b) stresses the importance of being open to including different ethnographic methods so as to capture life in motion. Analytically, this has meant that we have aimed for a constructive and creative research environment and done so by experimenting, early in the process, with writing, data collection, and theoretical influences (Back, 2007). This approach has also allowed us to adjust our approaches to the field as well as to critically reflect upon our conclusions and interpretations.

When analyzing our empirical material, we focused on the participants' perception of PIEDs in relation to their self-understanding, but also on the cultural framing of this practice and how doping use was understood in relation to different tendencies in the changeable fitness culture and gender order. The quotations and observations we present in the chapters have thus been selected for their ability to capture and describe both the subjective and the embodied experiences of PIEDs, diverse fitness doping trajectories and the gender regimen in which doping practice is constituted. In this sense, and although the analysis is mainly based on a narrative approach to the empirical material, we concur with Bourdieu and Wacquant (1992), who suggest that personal narratives must be situated within a wider social and cultural context if they are to be fully understood (see also Skeggs, 1997; Sparkes & Smith, 2007).

As researchers conducting research, we enter into personal and moral relationships, and our goal of advancing knowledge should not harm participants in any way. When initiating our longitudinal ethnographic study, we initially provided general information about our project to potential participants. Participants were informed of their right to pull out of the project at any time for any reason, with no questions asked. We were also careful to debrief the participants at the end of their participation, our goal being to inform them about the research outcomes and to identify any unforeseen harm, discomfort, or misconceptions. During the process of gathering and compiling the data, we made certain that names and other potential identifying details concerning the participants were omitted. Consequently, all names and places mentioned by participants have been anonymized to ensure confidentiality. Formal ethical approval was secured from the Regional Ethical Review Board of Linköping University before the study was initiated (Ref. No. 46-09).

Fitness Doping Netnography

In Chapter 6, and to some extent in Chapters 3, 7, and 8, we look at fitness doping in the context of online communication. Narratives published on the Internet are to be understood as quite a new source for empirical research, which mainly began as a field with the development of the Internet as a mass medium in the mid- to late 1990s (Hine, 2000; Hooley, Marriott, & Wellens, 2012). Due to the nature of the online social environment, this kind of research also seems to be continuously shifting.

In this project, we focused on the ways in which PIEDs were perceived and negotiated socially in the sociocultural context of the Internet-mediated, open online community, Flashback. On this platform, anybody with an Internet connection can read, learn about, and comment on their experience and knowledge of PIEDs. Basically, discussions on Flashback may concern 'just about anything,' but because the forum facilitates anonymous expression of opinions, there are many threads that concern prohibited activities. One popular theme is doping. There is also a subcategory to the doping theme called 'Course reports,' in which people present biographical reports on their first involvement with PIEDs and upload pictures of doping results. The information provided in this section gives us an idea of the demographics of the members of this community. While the personal information presented is limited, it would appear that many of the postings are made by young males. The age of the person behind a posting was seldom stated, however, but rather understood indirectly from the postings—for example, when a member discusses how to make time for daily training while still performing well in high school. Although there are some limitations regarding the age and gender of people who interact on Flashback, it is possible for anyone, regardless of gender and age, to create an account and engage in discussions on fitness doping. To deal with the gender 'bias' on Flashback, in Chapter 8 we chose to restrict our selection of postings to those explicitly stating that the poster was female.

When conducting the Internet study, our focus was 'on written accounts resulting from fieldwork studying the cultures and communities that emerge from online, computer mediated, or internet-based communications' (Kozinets, 2010, p. 58). We employed the method of netnography, sometimes also referred to as online ethnography, which was specifically designed for studying online communities. Developed by Kozinets (2010), netnography is methodologically indebted to the traditions and practices of ethnography and cultural anthropology (Hine, 2000). However, 'the field' being studied here is not typical and requires some clarifications: First, it cannot be neatly located to a certain place and community, which is a distinctive feature of more conventional ethnographies. Second, using mediated communication certainly limits our ability to gather all the information provided in, for example, face-to-face interaction and observations within any given culture. Third, using virtual methods also makes it nearly impossible for us to capture what is going on 'off the screen' (Hooley et al., 2012). However, regardless of these limitations, this type of material also has many similarities with more 'conventional' empirical sampling (Fleischmann, 2004; Sheehan, 2010). Social media, such as online communities, Facebook, and Twitter, are usually thematized in ways likely to attract and target specific audiences and lifestyle groups (Orgad, 2006). They can therefore be viewed as embedded in specific sociocultural and/or national contexts. Moreover, technological and social practices on the Internet have also meant that personal and community data have become more open and easier to access than ever before, thus creating a new form of intimacy (Joinson, McKenna, & Postmes, 2007). Naturally, this also affects people's everyday life and their relation to their cultural surroundings. Kozinets (2010) states:

The way in which technology and culture interact is a complex dance – an interweaving and intertwining. This element of technocultural change is present in our public spaces, our workplaces, our homes, our relationships, and our bodies – each institutional element intermixed with every other one. Technology constantly shapes and reshapes our bodies, our places, and our identities, and is shaped to our needs as well. (p. 22)

In the study, we focused on texts and images on Flashback, taking the perspective that these Internet communications and communities can, in one way or another, be viewed as cultural manifestations (Kozinets, 2010; Porter, 1997). Using different postings, we looked at how members of the Flashback community conceptualize and understand the use of PIEDs as an integral part of their everyday lives.

There are ethical issues associated with studying online communities. For instance, members may not expect their comments to be discussed and analyzed by researchers outside their community, which raises questions about consent and degrees of publicity (Walther, 2002). At the same time, however, it is reasonable to assume that any 'person who uses publicly available communication systems on the internet must be aware that these systems are, at their foundation and by definition, mechanisms for the storage, transmission, and retrieval of comments' (Walther, 2002, p. 207). The current status of Flashback is that the discussions presented are accessible to anyone with an Internet connection. Based on this and on the fact that the members use fictitious names in the community, one could argue that their personal privacy is not violated when they are quoted (Grodzinsky & Tavani, 2010; Rosenberg, 2010). There are, however, some aspects of the study that call for an extensive ethical concern for community members whose postings are used and analyzed. For example, we know that the members are engaged in a community where a criminalized activity is being discussed and often promoted. This means that use of excerpts could have legal repercussions, if the authorities were to locate the IP address of a particular member. Moreover, it was not always possible to find information regarding the age of a particular member, meaning that we did not know if participants were minors or adults.

To protect the identity of the community members on Flashback, the following measures were taken to secure confidentiality. First, fictitious user names were used. Second, the original postings were in Swedish and were subsequently translated to English for the book, making it harder for anyone to use available search engine technology to trace a particular posting. Third, when selecting excerpts, we have been careful not to focus on the most sensitive information given and have restricted our use of excerpts to those that promote relevant analysis (Hsiung, 2000). Omitted postings of relevance are discussed in the running text. Formal ethical approval to carry out this study was secured from the Regional Ethical Review Board of Linköping University (Ref. No. 2017/469-31).

National Comparative Study

Our investigation of two national cases, presented in Chapter 3, is based on empirical data in the form of interview and Internet material, research on fitness doping, and readings of secondary literature. This study was conducted in collaboration with an American researcher, April Dawn Henning, currently working at the University of Stirling, UK. The aim of contextualizing fitness doping using a national comparative analysis was to investigate how fitness doping can be understood in relation to different national and local contexts, where Sweden and the USA served as two cases representing different welfare state regimes.

Structuring the results for this chapter, we were inspired by Hall and Jefferson (1976), who identify three central nodes or analytical levels: structures, biographies, and cultures. We modified these to suit our study (and Chapter 3). *Structures* were used to discuss the formation of anti-doping policy and how policymakers in the two countries, over the past 40 years, have dealt with fitness doping as a social issue to be addressed through legislation. *Biographies* helped us study individual narratives and how doping trajectories are formed and connected to policy and to the formation of a bodybuilding community within gym and fitness culture (a discussion also developed elsewhere in the book). When it comes to the final level, *cultures,* we explored the symbolic landscape of the current preventative work being done in the two selected countries.

The rationale for choosing the two national case studies of Sweden and the USA was related to the research interests and nationality of the two authors. More importantly, however, Sweden and the USA represent two different kinds of welfare states. In our view, analyzing the different national approaches to fitness doping may, first, offer insights into national characteristics when it comes to prohibition, the presence (or absence) of preventative work, and more. Second, the case study approach may offer insights into fitness doping in relation to glocal processes through variability and the principle of comparative methodology.

The case study on fitness doping in the USA builds on an analysis of US drug and anti-doping policies and mainstream and niche media coverage of fitness doping. While not an exhaustive account of fitness media, the chosen examples presented in this case nevertheless highlight views within and outside the fitness community in the USA. The case study on fitness doping in Sweden was based on data gathered in the longitudinal ethnographic study and the netnographic study described previously in this chapter.

As regards data selection, the web pages and niche media examined were mainly selected strategically based partly on volume of readers and partly on analytical and theoretical relevance. Accordingly, the aim of our selection strategy, in addition to sampling popular bodybuilding Web sites, was to ensure that the chosen sites reflected different aspects and representations of glocal fitness doping. Our selection of individual postings on forums, biographies gathered through interviews, and policy documents followed the same logic.

References

Agar, M. (1996). *Professional stranger: Informal Introduction to ethnography*. London: Emerald Group.

Anderson-Levitt, K. (2006). Ethnography. In J. Green, G. Camilli, & P. Elmore (Eds.), *Handbook of complementary methods in education research* (pp. 279–296). Mahwah, NJ: Lawrence Erlbaum.

Andreasson, J., & Johansson, T. (2014). *The global gym: Gender, health and pedagogies*. Basingstoke, UK: Palgrave Macmillan.

Andreasson, J., & Johansson, T. (2019). *Extreme sports, extreme bodies: Gender, identities and bodies in motion*. Basingstoke, UK: Palgrave Macmillan.

Back, L. (2007). *The art of listening*. Oxford and New York: Berg Publishers.

Back, L. (2012a). Live sociology: Social research and its futures. *The Sociological Review, 60*(1), 18–39.

Back, L. (2012b). Tape recorder. In C. Lury & N. Wakeford (Eds.), *Inventive methods: The happening of the social*. London: Routledge.

Bourdieu, P., & Wacquant, L. (1992). *An invitation to reflexive sociology*. Cambridge: Polity Press.

Fangen, K. (2005). *Deltagande observation* [Participant observation]. Malmö: Liber.

Fleischmann, A. (2004). Narratives published on the Internet by parents of children with autism: What do they reveal and why is it important? *Focus on Autism and Other Developmental Disabilities, 19*(1), 35–43.

Geertz, C. (1973). Thick description: Toward an interpretive theory of culture. In *The interpretation of cultures: Selected essays* (pp. 3–30). New York: Basic Books.

Giddens, A. (1986). *The constitution of society*. Berkeley and Los Angeles: University of California Press.

Gratton, C., & Jones, I. (2004). *Research methods for sport studies*. London: Routledge.

Grodzinsky, F., & Tavani, H. (2010). Applying the 'contextual integrity' model of privacy to personal blogs in the blogosphere. *International Journal of Internet Research Ethics, 3*(1), 38–47.

Hall, S., & Jefferson, T. (Eds.). (1976). *Resistance through rituals*. London, UK: Hutchinson.

Hallqvist, A., & Hydén, L.-C. (2012). Work transition as told: A narrative approach to biographical learning. *Studies in Continuing Education, 35*(1), 1–16.

Hammersley, M., & Atkinson, P. (1995). *Ethnography: Principles in practice*. London: Routledge.

Hine, C. M. (2000). *Virtual ethnography*. London: Sage.

Hooley, T., Marriott, J., & Wellens, J. (2012). *What is online research?* New York: Bloomsbury.

Hsiung, R. C. (2000). The best of both worlds: An online self-help group hosted by a mental health professional. *Cyber Psychology & Behavior, 3*(6), 935–950.

Joinson, A., McKenna, K., & Postmes, T. (2007). *Oxford handbook of Internet psychology*. Oxford, UK: Oxford University Press.

Kozinets, R. (2010). *Netnography: Doing ethnographic research online*. London: Sage.

Lalander, P. (2003). *Hooked on heroin: Drugs and drifters in a globalized world.* Oxford and New York: Berg Publishers.

Merill, B., & West, L. (2009). *Using biographical methods in social research.* London: Sage.

Orgad, S. (2006). The cultural dimension of online communication: A study of breast cancer patients' Internet spaces. *New Media & Society, 8*(2), 877–899.

Pink, S. (2009). *Doing sensory ethnography.* London: Sage.

Porter, D. (1997). *Internet culture.* New York: Routledge.

Rosenberg, A. (2010). Virtual world research ethics and the private/public distinction. *International Journal of Internet Research Ethics, 3*(1), 23–37.

Salganik, M., & Heckathorn, D. (2004). Sampling and estimation in hidden populations using respondent-drive sampling. *Sociological Methodology, 34,* 193–239.

Shamir, B., Daya-Horesh, H., & Adler, D. (2005). Leading by biography: Towards a life-story approach to the study of leadership. *Leadership, 1*(1), 13–29.

Sheehan, K. B. (2010). Online research methodology: Reflections and speculations. *Journal of Interactive Advertising, 3*(1), 56–61.

Skeggs, B. (1997). *Formations of class and gender: Becoming respectable.* London: Sage.

Sparkes, A. C., & Smith, B. (2007). Narrative constructionist inquiry. In J. A. Holstein & J. F. Gubrium (Eds.), *Handbook of constructionist research* (pp. 295–314). New York: The Guilford Press.

Thurmond, V. A. (2001). The point of triangulation. *Journal of Nursing Scholarship, 33*(3), 253–258.

Walther, J. (2002). Research ethics in Internet-enabled research: Human subjects issues and methodological myopia. *Ethics and Information Technology, 4,* 205–216.

Index

© The Editor(s) (if applicable) and The Author(s),
under exclusive license to Springer Nature Switzerland AG 2020
J. Andreasson and T. Johansson, *Fitness Doping*,
https://doi.org/10.1007/978-3-030-22105-8